100 Questions & Answers About Eating Disorders

Carolyn Costin, LMFT, MA, MEd
Monte Nido Residential Center
Malibu, California

JONES AND BARTLETT PUBLISHERS
Sudbury, Massachusetts
BOSTON   TORONTO   LONDON   SINGAPORE

World Headquarters

Jones and Bartlett
Publishers
40 Tall Pine Drive
Sudbury, MA 01776
978-443-5000
info@jbpub.com
www.jbpub.com

Jones and Bartlett
Publishers Canada
6339 Ormindale Way
Mississauga, Ontario L5V 1J2
CANADA

Jones and Bartlett
Publishers International
Barb House, Barb Mews
London W6 7PA
UK

Jones and Bartlett's books and products are available through most bookstores and online booksellers. To contact Jones and Bartlett Publishers directly, call 800-832-0034, fax 978-443-8000, or visit our website, www.jbpub.com.

Substantial discounts on bulk quantities of Jones and Bartlett's publications are available to corporations, professional associations, and other qualified organizations. For details and specific discount information, contact the special sales department at Jones and Bartlett via the above contact information or send an email to specialsales@jbpub.com.

Production Credits
Executive Publisher: Christopher Davis
Associate Editor: Kathy Richardson
Production Director: Amy Rose
Production Editor: Tracey Chapman
Senior Marketing Manager: Katrina Gosek
Associate Marketing Manager: Rebecca Wasley
Manufacturing and Inventory Coordinator: Amy Bacus
Composition: Judith Webb
Cover Design: Kate Ternullo
Cover Image: © Photos.com,© Vova Pomortzeff/Shutterstock, Inc. © Paul B. Moor/Shutterstock, Inc.
Printing and Binding: Malloy, Inc.
Cover Printing: Malloy, Inc.

Library of Congress Cataloging-in-Publication Data
Costin, Carolyn.
100 questions & answers about eating disorders / Carolyn Costin. — 1st ed.
  p. cm.
Includes bibliographical references and index.
ISBN-13: 978-0-7637-4500-4 (pbk.)
ISBN-10: 0-7637-4500-6 (pbk.)
1. Eating disorders—Miscellanea. I. Title. II. Title: One hundred questions and answers about eating disorders.
RC552.E18C667 2007
616.85'26—dc22

                                                                20060379696048
6048
Printed in the United States of America
11 10 09 08 07   10 9 8 7 6 5 4 3 2 1

CONTENTS

Questions 1-24 discuss the different types of eating disorders and the signs for recognizing an eating disorder, including:
- What is an eating disorder?
- Is it true that exercise can be a form of purging?
- How common are eating disorders?

Questions 25-34 describe different medical issues, including:
- What are the medical complications involved in eating disorders?
- How do I know if I need a bone density test?
- My teeth are eroding. Is this from purging and is there anything I can do?

Questions 35-44 discuss the causes of an eating disorder, including:
- I often hear that eating disorders are all about control. Is this true?
- Does the media cause eating disorders?
- Do psychological problems cause eating disorders?

Questions 45-62 describe options for getting help, including:
- If I think I have an eating disorder, what should I do?
- How do I choose a good therapist?
- Do I need to see a nutritionist?

This is a little book about a big topic, so big that it could take volumes to answer all the questions you as a reader might have. A book like this could even be written for each eating disorder diagnosis. But this book is meant to be a quick guide. It is geared for the person who needs to find simple, helpful answers to big, complicated problems and questions. It is meant to help lead you to further resources who or which can then provide more detailed and specific understanding and help for your particular situation. I hope this book whets your appetite (pun intended) to learn more. Perhaps it will even get others of you to seek help.

Having an eating disorder can be complicated, frustrating, confusing, and scary. The field of eating disorder treatment is relatively new, and we are continuing to gain a better understanding of these **biopsychosocial** illnesses. (Throughout this book, a word presented in **bold type** is defined in the Glossary.) I wish a book like this one had existed when I developed my own eating disorder, anorexia nervosa, as a young teen. I wish my parents had been able to read such a book.

I use an informal tone in the book, as if I am answering questions from someone sitting in my living room. There will be many questions left unanswered; therefore throughout the book I refer readers to other sources to find details on things I briefly discuss. You will notice that I rarely use the word "patient" and more often use the word "client." I prefer client, and this is what I use in my practice. However, various professionals prefer otherwise, so I use both in this book and in all of my writings. Another thing I always try to do when writing, lecturing at conferences, or talking to clients and their families is avoid using the terms "anorexic," "bulimic," or "binge eater." I prefer to think of and refer to my clients and others with eating disorders as people who *suffer* from anorexia, bulimia, or binge eating disorder. I want my clients to think of themselves in this way also. I believe this helps keep them from overly identifying with the illness. They are not the illness; they are people who *have* the illness. As you will see I also believe they can be recovered from these illnesses. Additionally, I prefer the shortened commonly used way of describing these illnesses. Therefore the more cumbersome "anorexia nervosa" becomes "anorexia." I write pretty much like I talk. In many ways, my clients have written much of this book. Clients whom I am currently treating and those from the past continue to find their way onto the pages of anything I write. They show up in what they have taught me and what I pass on here to you. They show up in case material, as I have taken excerpts directly from sessions with them, disguising them so as not to be recognizable. Finally, the clients show up in their own written words, as I have used a few of their journal entries to personalize some of the material.

In writing this book, I use many resources in the field and have gleaned information from prominent researchers, but the flavor and tone is definitely mine as my opinions are scattered throughout the manuscript. They are informed opinions derived from the quantity and quality of information that comes directly from my personal experience. My own battle and subsequent recovery from anorexia nervosa during the early 1970s and my experiences as an eating disorder therapist since 1977 add a strong personal influence. I am not a researcher, but I have probably clocked more hours of individual eating disorder therapy than anyone on the planet. I thank my clients and their families for all the lessons learned, joys shared, and growth that has taken place in all of us over these many years. Every client I have seen has helped me to help the next one that comes along and the next and many more to come.

I thank my husband, Bruce, for allowing my late nights and early mornings with clients. I thank my parents, brother, and sister for loving me through my eating disorder and being wonderful human beings. I thank my friends for being who they are and just being there. I thank my colleagues all over the world who share in this battle against eating disorders and those who are spending their lives to prevent them.

I don't believe we will eradicate eating disorders in my lifetime, but I do believe we need to continue to try. We did not always live in a world in which what you weigh is more important than who you are; schools give body fat report cards, liposuction is a form of weight loss, emaciated models walk the fashion runways, children vomit to lose weight, and eating disorder treatment centers are the fastest growing type of mental health facilities. We do not need to continue to live in this kind of world. I ask my clients what will future generations think when they look back at us? Will "size one" jeans be compared with Chinese foot binding of the past, which we now consider torture? What will they think when they see images of emaciated fashion models who get paid thousands of dollars a day to walk down the runways with their unhealthy bodies, while at the same time other females of the exact age, height, and weight are paying thousands of dollars to be treated for anorexia? I hope we can change this trend so that future generations will see that we realized it was terribly wrong and fixed it. I still believe we can, but it will require us all to wake up and begin to nurture what really counts, to turn the cliché "it's what's inside that counts" into a reality. I work at this every day and hope that you, my dear reader, because you have some interest in this topic, will begin to do so, too.

Carolyn Costin, LMFT, MA, MEd
Malibu, California

I am blessed to have found my calling. My work is challenging but rewarding and has an impact on people's lives. I love working with eating disorder clients, their families, and significant others. I have spent all my adult life and a good part of my adolescent years immersed in eating disorders, from the ages of 15 to 22 as a sufferer of anorexia nervosa and from 23 onward recovered and treating others who suffered from these illnesses. Since I recovered I had no doubt that everyone else could become recovered also, and this has proven invaluable in my treatment success. I grew up alongside the field of eating disorders and have watched as both the number of people with eating disorders has increased as well as the number of treatment professionals, programs, and philosophies to treat them.

Eating disorders are devastating illnesses and need to be recognized as such. It has taken a long time, but the public and professionals alike seem to be getting the message that eating disorders are not just diets gone bad or rich white girls acting out. Still there are many misconceptions that I continue to encounter, such as "if you look normal and your weight is normal, you don't have an eating disorder," "if you purge, you have bulimia," or "eating disorders are all about control and attention"; the newest one is the belief that "eating disorders are solely caused by genetics." I hope to dispel these and other myths in this book.

I can think of 1,000 questions I would like to answer about eating disorders, but 900 of them will have to be saved for other writings, lectures, or workshops. Most people who know me know that I have a lot to say about the subject. After 30 years of working in the field in a variety of ways and settings, I have learned much that I can share with others. Starting in the late 1970s as a private practice therapist, I cut my teeth working alone on case after case of individuals showing up with anorexia, bulimia, and binge eating or some variation of these illnesses. I found no books to help me and no mentors to learn from, although both of these eventually came along. In these early years, I developed a style of working with eating disorders that I still use today, the concept that everyone has an eating disorder self and a healthy self and that healing takes place when these two parts of self can be integrated. Therefore underlying all my treatment methods, strategies, and interventions is the belief that I must strengthen each person's healthy self so that it can be in charge. The idea is not to get rid of the eating disorder self but to understand that this part of a person's psyche is meant to be a guide, an alarm system if you will, that alerts the healthy self to pain and problems but should not try to take care of them with eating disorder behaviors as it once learned to do.

This is a hopeful way to look at eating disorders as illnesses and at human beings with problems in general. This way has worked, and today I am grateful to have experienced the full recovery of countless individuals who suffered from every possible form of eating disorder one can imagine. I have seen 8-year-old girls starving themselves to death because they fear getting too fat; a 65-year-old woman with a collapsed colon from too many laxatives, such that she had to be attached to a bag to deal with her fecal matter; a young man with bulimia who chose to have an eating disorder to distract himself and his parents from something more difficult to face, his homosexuality. I have seen identical twins where both have anorexia, where one has anorexia and the other bulimia, and where one has an eating disorder and the other does not. I saw one case in which one twin had anorexia and the other had binge eating disorder up until college when the situation reversed and each twin developed the other twin's disorder. It was almost as if their combined weight had to always remain the same. I have seen people who have suffered the most egregious forms of abuse, and consequently had the most severe eating disorders, get better and become fully recovered. I have also seen cases early on, where there were no other diagnoses or complications, and there was a good support system and yet the illness dragged on and on and became chronic. People die from eating disorders, and this should not have to be the case. I hope that with all our future efforts, soon no more will succumb.

This book offers answers to many of the commonly asked questions I get from the public, from those with eating disorders, from their loved ones, and from professionals. I provide an overview of what these illnesses are, the various problems that cause them, and the myriad of problems they cause. Well-supported suggestions for when, how, and why to get better are all included here. Hopefully family members and significant others will learn ways to approach and better cope with these illnesses and will be better prepared when seeking help for loved ones.

I provide an overview of what kind of treatment is available and what to expect from different treatment professionals. There are various philosophical approaches to treating these disorders, and a brief description will help readers get acquainted with them. I shed light on what happens behind the closed doors of therapy rooms in individual, group, and family therapy and describe for readers how nutritionists can fit into an overall treatment plan. I also share what can be done if treatment on an outpatient basis is not working. It can be daunting to try to figure out all the available options, so I delineate these in a simple fashion and help readers see how these alternatives can be helpful. Alternative treatments are also increasingly being sought for eating disorders, and I introduce readers to those most commonly used with eating disorders today. Finally, I speak of prevention and give readers some tips on how to get involved in this important effort.

I hope this book serves not only as a guide but as a motivator for someone to get help, to help another, or even to do something to help us all begin to prevent eating disorders and body image dissatisfaction so prevalent in the culture we live in today.

PART ONE

Overview of Eating Disorders

What is an eating disorder?

What is the difference between
anorexia nervosa and bulimia nervosa?

I binge but do not purge.
Is that considered an eating disorder?

More...

1. What is an eating disorder?

Eating disorders almost always start out as diets, but these disorders are not just about food and weight.

An eating disorder is an illness that manifests itself in a variety of unhealthy eating and weight control habits that become obsessive, compulsive, and/or impulsive in nature. Eating disorders almost always start out as diets, but these disorders are not just about food and weight. Individuals who have eating disorders also tend to suffer from issues of self-worth, depression, anxiety, or some other psychological symptoms. Medical complications are also demonstrated in these disorders, ranging from hypothermia and hair loss to esophageal rupture. Eating disorders are currently understood as having multiple causes, including genetic, biological, psychological, and cultural. The three main types of eating disorders are anorexia nervosa, bulimia nervosa, and binge eating disorder (BED). The first two are listed in the *Diagnostic and Statistical Manual of Mental Disorders*, 4th edition (text revision) *(DSM-IV-TR)*. BED, which has the distinct feature of not being associated with compensatory weight loss behaviors, is not yet considered a separate illness but is included in the *DSM-IV-TR* as one of several eating disorder variants listed in another diagnostic catch-all category, **Eating Disorders Not Otherwise Specified (EDNOS)**. This category includes syndromes that resemble anorexia nervosa or bulimia nervosa but fall short of an essential feature or symptom duration, thus precluding either diagnosis. Also in the EDNOS category are eating disorders that may present quite differently from anorexia nervosa or bulimia nervosa, such as BED. Binge eating disorder is also listed in Appendix B of the *DSM-IV-TR* as one of several proposals that were suggested for possible inclusion as a diagnostic category.

To understand the various eating disorders, it helps to see the diagnostic criteria as taken directly from the *DSM-IV-TR*. Case examples are also helpful.

The *DSM-IV-TR* Diagnostic Criteria for 307.1 Anorexia Nervosa

A. Refusal to maintain body weight at or above a minimally normal weight for age and height (e.g., weight loss leading to maintenance of body weight less than 85% of that expected or failure to make expected weight gain during period of growth, leading to body weight less than 85% of that expected).

B. Intense fear of gaining weight or becoming fat, even though underweight.

C. Disturbance in the way in which one's body weight or shape is experienced, undue influence of body weight or shape on self-evaluation, or denial of the seriousness of the current low body weight.

D. In postmenarcheal females, amenorrhea (i.e., the absence of at least three consecutive menstrual cycles). (A woman is considered to have amenorrhea if her periods occur only after following hormone, e.g., estrogen, administration.)

Restricting Type: During the current episode of anorexia nervosa, the person has not regularly engaged in binge eating or purging behavior (i.e., self-induced vomiting or the misuse of laxatives, diuretics, or enemas).

Binge Eating/Purging Type: During the current episode of anorexia nervosa, the person has regularly engaged in binge eating or purging behavior (i.e., self-induced vomiting or the misuse of laxatives, diuretics, or enemas).

The following case examples show the diversity of clients in the anorexia nervosa diagnostic category. This is important to dispel stereotypes that are often associated with this illness.

Case Example 1, Jill: Jill is a 16-year-old white adolescent, who is the star of her high school track team. Her mother brought her to see me because of significant recent weight loss. Jill also had become a vegetarian and often would skip meals, saying she had already eaten or would eat later. Because she was an excellent student and had never been a problem, Jill's parents let things go on for too long. Jill was now moody and irritable and looked extremely thin. In fact, a recent weigh-in at the doctor's office revealed she was 102 lbs. at her 5'8" height. I also discovered that she was no longer menstruating. Her periods had stopped about a year ago, but she did not think much of it because other girls on her track team also no longer menstruated. She had not told her parents this information. Jill was pleasant and somewhat reserved and stated that although she thought she looked fine, she knew she probably needed to gain some weight because of her parents and the doctor. However, she was not sure she had an eating disorder. When looking over a food inventory I had her keep for a few days, it revealed that she was eating approximately 900 calories a day. She was reluctant to add more when it was suggested. Jill denied any laxative use, vomiting, or other forms of purging but did seem to exercise to excess even though she was on the track team. Jill did more than the regular required workouts.
Jill meets the criteria for anorexia nervosa, restricting type.

Case Example 2, Ali: Ali is a 40-year-old, part Asian, married woman with two children. She spent her early years in Japan with an American mother and a Japanese father. She was on and off diets as a teenager and used various dieting methods. She had even tried purging a few times by vomiting, and there were several instances where she had taken laxatives. Her weight had remained fairly normal over the years, with the exception of an episode in college in which she lost several pounds but put them back on with pressure from her parents. Now grown with a husband and two children and a full-time job as a teacher, Ali came to see me because of the current stress in her life. She reported that her husband had threatened to leave and she was coming to therapy to save her marriage. She was emaciated and frail. Ali reported a weight loss of 25 pounds over the last 6 or 7 months (she was not exactly sure). She said the weight loss was due to stress and that she had a hard time sleeping. She also admitted the occasional use of laxatives because she was frequently constipated and so they were necessary. When pressed for details on all her dieting and weight loss behaviors she did not report vomiting. However, when asked specifically if she ever purged by vomiting, she admitted that occasionally when she ate certain foods or too much she would "get sick." When asked if this meant vomiting, she replied, "Yes." She reported that sometimes when she ate too much she considered it a binge, but it was unclear how much food she actually ate during these episodes, and she did not want to share further details about it. When asked about menstruation Ali said she was not sure when she had her period last, but with prompting it was clear that it had been a few months at least but that it was always irregular even as a kid, so she did not notice. Ali had not been to a doctor to discuss her weight loss, constipation, or insomnia. Ali said she was 5'4" and did not know what she weighed. I sent her to a doctor for a physical, who confirmed her height and reported her weight at 86 pounds.

*Ali also meets the criteria for **anorexia nervosa** but of the **binge eating/purge type**.*

Case Example 3, Kevin: Kevin is a 9-year-old boy who was brought to me by his mother when his weight had dropped approximately 20 pounds. At 5 feet tall and approximately 87 pounds he looked skinny and frail but had a great deal of energy. Kevin seemed to be anxious and preoccupied during the assessment but was cooperative. I discovered from Kevin and his mother that Kevin had been cutting back on foods ever since his father had a heart attack and had begun dieting. Kevin noticed his father cutting back on fat and desserts, reading labels, and exercising for the first time in his life. There was a lot of talk in the family regarding nutrition and health. Kevin took it seriously and at first was praised by his family for following his father's good eating habits. When it was noticed that Kevin was losing weight, his mother tried to talk to him. She decided to pack his lunch for him instead of letting him pack it, but Kevin threw away the cookies and chips when he was at school. Kevin lost more weight, and his father stepped in and tried to discipline him and make him eat. Kevin's dad could usually get him to eat dinner, but was gone during the day due to work. Kevin pretended to eat his breakfast but often was able to hide much of it in his napkin or backpack. The more breakfast he ate, the more of his lunch he threw away at school. Kevin became terrified of gaining any weight and continued to lose weight in spite of his assurance to his parents that he would not lose any more. Kevin also talked about being fat and looking fat all the time. He was obsessed with body fat and wanted to have his body fat tested and cried when his mother refused. When his mom took Kevin to the family doctor, she was advised to take Kevin for a consultation with someone trained in eating disorders. Kevin meets the criteria for **anorexia nervosa, restricting type.**

Overview of Eating Disorders

The *DSM-IV-TR* Diagnostic Criteria for 307.51 Bulimia Nervosa

A. Recurrent episodes of binge eating. An episode of binge eating is characterized by both of the following:

1. Eating, in a discreet period of time (e.g., within any 2-hour period), an amount of food that is definitely larger than most people would eat during a similar period of time and under similar circumstances.

2. A sense of lack of control over eating during the episode (e.g., a feeling that one cannot stop eating or control what or how much one is eating).

B. Recurrent inappropriate compensatory behavior in order to prevent weight gain, such as self-induced vomiting; misuse of laxatives, diuretics, enemas, or other medications; fasting; or excessive exercise.

C. The binge eating and other inappropriate compensatory behaviors both occur, on average, at least twice a week for 3 months.

D. Self-evaluation is unduly influenced by body shape and weight.

E. The disturbance does not occur exclusively during episodes of anorexia nervosa.

Purging Type: During the current episode of bulimia nervosa, the person has regularly engaged in self-induced vomiting or the misuse of laxatives, diuretics, or enemas.

Nonpurging Type: During the current episode of bulimia nervosa, the person has used other inappropriate compensatory behaviors, such as fasting or excessive exercise, but has not regularly engaged in self-induced vomiting or the misuse of laxatives, diuretics, or enemas.

Bulimia nervosa is an illness that presents itself in a wide variety of ways. The following examples are just three of many possible presentations.

Case Example 1, Henna: Henna, a 30-year old, married, white woman, came to my treatment center, Monte Nido, for an evaluation for residential care. She was a bright, articulate, career woman who had a history of both drug use and eating problems. She had recently completed treatment for drug and alcohol abuse but upon returning home could not get her binging and purging under control. She had continued her bulimia while in the drug treatment program, but the staff had not noticed because she hid it very well. Now without her drugs she felt out of control, and all kinds of painful images of a past sexual abuse were emerging. Henna found herself binging and purging three to four times a day and could not work or even get herself to therapy appointments. According to her treatment records, Henna was approximately 5'6" and 230 pounds. Henna was obsessed with her weight and thought about losing weight most of her waking hours. Sometimes she believed that if she did not lose weight, she would not be able to live in her body. Henna's husband said that he had no idea the eating disorder was that bad, but because the drugs and alcohol were gone he thought perhaps she was using this now more than ever to cope. Henna seemed very motivated for treatment and believed the last piece of work she had to do to really get well and lead a healthy life was to get rid or her eating disorder. Henna meets the criteria for **bulimia nervosa/purging type.**

Case Example 2, Shannon: Shannon is an 18-year-old teenager from Ireland who was out of control. By the time I first saw her she had crashed her car, gotten a D.U.I. (driving *under the influence) citation, stolen her parents' credit cards, dropped out of school, died her hair orange, and gotten several tattoos and piercings. Her voice was raspy from the amount of vomiting she did and cigarettes she smoked, which were, incidentally, the same amount, about 15 times a day. She had a bad case of reflux, but medication was only partly helpful. Shannon had been to two other treatment centers and had seen several therapists and psychiatrists. She was taking five medications but had no idea if any of them helped. At one point she was diagnosed with **attention deficit disorder**, but when she got caught selling her medication to her peers and snorting it with them, her psychiatrist refused to prescribe more. Her parents also told her they would not pay for it. She came for an assessment for residential or day treatment—she did not seem to care either way—but her parents wanted her in 24-hour care. Shannon's parents were beside themselves and really wanted her to get help this time and stick with the treatment; however, they were not very insistent or firm with her in the session. Shannon had left all previous treatments too early and had either not been helped or had relapsed. When asked what would be different this time, Shannon reported, "…I am sick of this illness and all the crap that goes with it and I'm just really ready to get better."*

*Shannon meets the diagnostic criteria for **bulimia nervosa/purging type**.*

Case Example 3, Eric: Eric is a 20-year-old athlete and an excellent runner and swimmer. In fact, he was just beginning to develop his biking skills and become a triathlete when he first came to see me. He is attractive and for most of his life had lots of friends and girlfriends. Aside from wanting to be a triathlete, he wants to be a chiropractor and studies health. He had become increasingly health conscious over the years and had gotten his body fat down to almost nothing, around 5%. Eric also had increased his workouts such that he

ADHD

Attention deficit hyperactivity disorder (ADHD, and sometimes referred to as ADD) is thought by some but not all to be a neurological disorder, usually diagnosed in childhood, which manifests itself with symptoms such as hyperactivity, forgetfulness, poor impulse control, and distractibility.

had hardly any time for his friends; in fact, over the last few years several girlfriends had left him, complaining of his selfishness and his obsession with exercise. He came to see me on the pleading of his girlfriend, with whom he was in love and wanted to marry. His coach had also become concerned about Eric's eating habits and overall health. Eric never took rest days, frequently went on fasts, and was getting injured frequently and not performing as well. Both the coach and the girlfriend came to the first appointment and discussed their concerns. Eric would probably not have come otherwise. I saw Eric for 3 months before he admitted that he secretly binged on food late at night, several times a week, and believed it had gotten completely out of hand. He said he tried purging by vomiting, but it was too difficult and made him feel too bad physically, which was the reason he exercised beyond the coach's recommendations and could never take rest days. He had also tried diet pills. Eric said he had gotten some ideas a couple of years prior from reading the book, Seabiscutt, which discusses methods that jockeys use to lose weight. He was afraid of gaining weight and ruining his physique and his triathlon chances, but he could not stop eating. The food rituals had become longer and longer, sometimes going hours into the night, and this caused him to also suffer from lack of sleep. After finally telling the truth about all his symptoms, Eric was relieved and began to work in therapy.

*Eric meets the criteria for **bulimia nervosa, nonpurging type**.*

The *DSM-IV-TR* Diagnostic Criteria for 307.50 Eating Disorders Not Otherwise Specified

The Eating Disorders Not Otherwise Specified (EDNOS) category is for disorders of eating that do not meet the criteria for any specific eating disorder. Examples include:

1. For females, all of the criteria for anorexia nervosa are met except that the individual has regular menses.

2. All of the criteria for anorexia nervosa are met except that, despite significant weight loss, the individual's current weight is in the normal range.

3. All of the criteria for bulimia nervosa are met except that the binge eating and inappropriate compensatory mechanisms occur at a frequency of less than twice a week or for a duration of less than 3 months.

4. The regular use of inappropriate compensatory behavior by an individual of normal body weight after eating small amounts of food (e.g., self-induces vomiting after the consumption of two cookies).

5. Repeatedly chewing and spitting out, but not swallowing, large amounts of food.

6. Binge eating disorder: Recurrent episodes of binge eating in the absence of the regular use of inappropriate compensatory behaviors characteristic of bulimia nervosa.

EDNOS is a category with numerous variations of disordered eating that do not meet the full criteria for anorexia or bulimia. Clients in this category can be very severe or they can have eating disorders that have not progressed to the full-blown diagnosis of anorexia or bulimia. Two such cases follow.

Case Example 1, Maggie: Maggie is an African American college student who was normal weight but constantly preoccupied with her weight and overall appearance. She dieted frequently and would even vomit occasionally after a big night out with friends, where she drank a bit too much. She never binged. The thought of it horrified her, and she swore she would never do that. Maggie had stopped getting

her period even though her weight of 112 was normal for her 5'3½" frame. She had skipped her period for about the last 3 months, but it had been irregular before that for about a year. She was constantly counting calories and found it difficult to eat anything with fat in it at all. She had become obsessed with fat when her father had gone on a very strict diet. Maggie would occasionally drink, but this was rare. She was becoming increasingly isolative because she did not want to go out for fear of having to face food. Even seeing others eat food was difficult. Her daily calories ranged from approximately 500 to 1,500, depending on the day. Her food choices had become very limited, with lots of frozen yogurt, protein bars, coffee drinks, salads, and occasional sushi. Maggie was tearful as she described a feeling of never being safe, not knowing what to eat, and not ever feeling comfortable in her body.
*Maggie meets the criteria for **EDNOS**.*

Case Example 2, Nate: Nate came to see me after he had lost 180 pounds. He was now only 165 pounds at a height of 5'10" but claimed he saw himself still as the 345-pound man he once had been. Nate had been an athlete, playing high school and college football, but always tended to be overweight and was not very good at his sport. After college Nate tried dieting, because his 345 pounds, helpful as a linebacker, was no longer practical. He also stopped working out and lost a good deal of muscle he had put on during training. Nate said he felt horrible and fat and disgusting. Nate lost a few pounds occasionally, only to gain them back. Nate was ashamed of his body and afraid he would never experience a long-term relationship. Eventually, Nate was approved for bypass surgery to help him lose weight. After the surgery Nate began losing weight but had become obsessed with it. He weighed himself several times a day and charted the results. Nate also had reduced his diet partly due to the recommendations by the nutritionist who saw him after the surgery. Nate, however, had taken the recommendations too far and had begun to exclude all kinds of food from his diet. By the time of our first visit Nate was eating about 600 calories a day and was unable to add new foods for fear of "gaining weight." Nate meets the criteria for EDNOS.

The *DSM-IV-TR* Research Criteria for Binge Eating Disorder

A. Recurrent episodes of binge eating. An episode of binge eating is characterized by both of the following:

   1. Eating, in a discrete period of time (e.g., within any 2-hour period), an amount of food that is definitely larger than most people would eat in a similar period of time under similar circumstances.

   2. A sense of lack of control over eating during the episode (e.g., a feeling that one cannot stop eating or control what or how much one is eating).

B. The binge eating episodes are associated with three (or more) of the following:

   1. Eating much more rapidly than normal.

   2. Eating until feeling uncomfortably full.

   3. Eating large amounts of food when not feeling physically hungry.

   4. Eating alone because of being embarrassed by how much one is eating.

   5. Feeling disgusted with oneself, depressed, or very guilty after overeating.

C. Marked distress regarding binge eating is present.

D. The binge eating occurs, on average, at least 2 days a week for 6 months.

Note: The method of determining frequency differs from that used for bulimia nervosa; future research should address whether the preferred method of setting a frequency threshold is counting the number of days on which binges occur or counting the number of episodes of binge eating.

E. The binge eating is not associated with the regular use of inappropriate compensatory behaviors (e.g., purging, fasting, excessive exercise) and does not occur exclusively during the course of anorexia nervosa or bulimia nervosa.

The following examples show binge eating in two very different age groups.

Case Example 1, Debbie: Debbie came to see me with her parents shortly after her 14th birthday. Debbie was overweight according to her pediatrician and needed help losing weight. Her parents had tried a dietitian, but Debbie hated her and refused to talk. The dietitian recommended they take her to see me. In my first few sessions Debbie acted like nothing was wrong and she did not understand why she had to see me. She said her weight was her parents' problem, not hers. I decided to not talk to her about her weight or eating habits, so we talked about a variety of other things, such as her interests, her parents, her school, and her peers. This led to her admission of being teased at school and to a discussion regarding her weight. I saw Debbie with her family sometimes and alone sometimes. I initially asked the parents to stop trying to control her food. After she had talked about the teasing, Debbie found it easier to discuss other difficult things. Eventually, she told me about her food stashes and how she got up late at night to eat whatever her parents did not want her to eat. She described spending her money on food after school and hiding this from her parents. Debbie described long binges that took place after school several times a week when she was alone at home. She believed these were out of control and she could not stop herself. Debbie agreed she had a problem but didn't want her parents to know this because she said it would give them too much satisfaction and she preferred for them to think she liked herself this way. Debbie meets the proposed criteria for **binge eating disorder***.*

Case Example 2, Jake: Jake is a 36-year-old Italian man who had been overweight his whole life. He had first been to obesity camp when he was 10 years old. No diet had ever worked for very long. Jake's mother was obese, and he had hated seeing her unhappy and depressed. He remembered watching as a child when people would tease her and she would cry. Jake swore he would never be like his mother. As Jake got older he stopped caring so much about how heavy he had become. He gave up dieting and started to go the opposite direction, eating whenever and whatever he wanted. He read books that said he needed to stop dieting and learn how to eat intuitively. So he did. He ate what he wanted, which was pasta and ice cream and bread and butter and cream sauce and cream pie and chocolate bars. He also ate a lot of it. Jake did not seem to know when he was hungry or full. To him it seemed like he was hungry or eating. Jake said he felt out of control around food, spending so much money on food he was going into debt. This caused Jake to continue to gain weight, and at his first appointment Jake had no idea what he weighed. He wanted to have some idea so we tried my scale, with his back to the number so he could not see it. The scale registered its full amount, 350 pounds, but we could not determine how much more he might weigh. Eventually, we found a horse scale on which to weigh Jake, and he weighed 450 pounds. Jake was serious about treatment. He knew he had an eating disorder besides being overweight, and he wanted treatment for it.
Jake meets the criteria for **binge eating disorder***.*

2. What is the difference between anorexia nervosa and bulimia nervosa?

Anorexia and bulimia are similar illnesses, and many people who suffer from one also develop the other. Approximately 50% of those with anorexia develop bulimia. Both illnesses are characterized by issues of excessive concern with weight and shape. Restricting food intake; binging and purging calories, for example, by vomiting or taking laxatives; and excessive exercise to burn calories are all found in both disorders. The main difference is that to be diagnosed with anorexia the individual must be underweight, which is 15% below expected weight for age and height, and, if a post menarcheal female, have amenorrhea. Individuals who binge and purge and others who do not binge but do purge are often misdiagnosed with bulimia even though they meet the weight loss and amenorrhea criteria for anorexia. These individuals should be diagnosed with anorexia, binge/purge type.

3. I binge but do not purge. Is that considered an eating disorder?

Binge eating is commonly discussed as the third main eating disorder, even though it does not have its own diagnostic category in the *DSM-IV-TR*. This disorder, formerly referred to as compulsive overeating, is still being researched and discussed to determine whether it warrants its own diagnostic category or whether it should remain in the category of EDNOS, where it is currently listed in the *DSM-IV-TR*. However, just because you binge does not mean you have this disorder. Many people have occasional eating splurges that they consider binges, but these people do not meet the criteria for BED. In fact, I have heard people with anorexia say they binge, but when asked for details they describe a few cookies or any "fatten-ing" food or eating late at night as a binge. It is important to understand what the word binge really means and what the other features for BED are. You should look at Question 1 and check the diagnostic criteria for this disorder to determine whether you have this illness.

4. Is it true that you can be a normal weight and still have an eating disorder?

People often make the mistake of thinking that if you have an eating disorder you look emaciated or overweight. In fact, you can be either of these and not have an eating disorder. There are a variety of reasons why people weigh what they do. Eating disorders are mental illnesses that involve a variety of features. A focus on weight and shape and weight control behaviors are certainly part of anorexia and bulimia, but the only actual weight criteria for any eating disorder is that for anorexia nervosa. To be officially diagnosed with this illness, you must be 15% below that expected for your age and height. All other eating disorders—bulimia nervosa, BED, and EDNOS—have no specific weight criteria necessary for the diagnosis.

5. If I only purge my meals but don't ever binge, do I have bulimia?

Often people think that if you purge, you must have bulimia. There are individuals who purge their food, through various methods, but do not binge. To be diagnosed with bulimia, an individual has to both binge and purge or compensate for the binge in some other way. Some people who purge also meet the criteria for anorexia, binge/purge type, but others are more appropriately diagnosed with EDNOS.

6. My doctor says I have EDNOS. Does that mean my eating disorder is not bad?

Many people believe that a diagnosis of EDNOS means that the individual has a less severe form of eating disorder. Sometimes this is the case, but not always. People very entrenched in a chronic eating disorder or with serious medical complications from their eating disorder are often diagnosed with EDNOS. For example, a person who meets all the criteria for anorexia but has not missed three consecutive periods can still be very ill, especially if she has been losing weight for many months or even years, as was the case of a person I treated who first had BED and then developed anorexia.

7. Is obesity an eating disorder?

Obesity is a medical illness, not a psychiatric illness like the eating disorders.

Obesity is a medical illness, not a psychiatric illness like the eating disorders. However, some obese people also meet the diagnostic criteria for BED or for bulimia. Studies are inconsistent, but data reported in Richard Gordon's book, *Eating Disorders: Anatomy of a Social Epidemic* (2000), revealed that as many as 30% of people in weight loss programs meet the criteria for BED. Additionally, not all people with BED are obese; a small number of individuals with BED are normal weight.

8. My 10-year-old daughter is a very picky eater. Is this an eating disorder?

Lots of kids are picky eaters, but most grow out of it and are not harmed. It is important to watch your child and see whether he or she is getting enough calories to gain weight and develop properly. If your child seems overly picky and the problem continues to get worse, go to a pediatrician to get professional advice on the matter. If you are unsatisfied, go to another. Some childhood eating problems that have not been described so far do not manifest with the preoccupation with weight and shape; these are selective eating (eating a very limited variety of foods), restrictive eating (eating minimal quantities of food), food phobia (fear of eating/swallowing specific food or foods, usually lumpy or solid foods), and food avoidance emotional disorder (food restriction is due to an emotional problem such as anxiety, sadness, or obsessionality, which interferes with appetite). If a child has one of these disorders, it is important to seek help. A good resource is *Eating Disorders, A Parents' Guide* (Bryant-Waugh and Lask, 2004).

9. Have eating disorders been around historically and for how long?

Eating disorders are not new. The Ancient Greeks were known to binge and purge, and the Romans during the time of Caesar (700 B.C.) were well known for their vomitoriums, which were built for the purpose of making it easy for them to engage in gluttony and then vomit to continue their consumption of food and drink. Obviously, this binge and purge ritual was not considered an illness. Selfinduced vomiting, recommended as a health practice in ancient Egypt, was also not considered an illness. Over-concern with thinness, a feature of bulimia, was not a part of these practices. Bulimia nervosa as we know it today was only officially added as a mental illness to the *Diagnostic and Statistical Manual of Mental Disorders*, 3rd edition (revised), in 1987.

Anorexia seems to have roots going back to the thirteenth century, when certain religious females were actually canonized as saints for their fasting practices. In his book, *Holy Anorexia*, Rudolf Bell (1985) describes these saints as "holy anorexics." Bell describes how in the self-denying search for purity and holiness, the saints starved themselves, were hyperactive and perfectionist, and lost an excess of 25% of their normal body weight. Some of these women were suspected of binge eating practices as well as restricting. This is strikingly familiar to individuals with anorexia today, except that today the self-denial is for thinness and self-control.

In the search for both holiness and thinness, the pursuit can become the goal. To be self-sacrificing, to be independent of needs, and to nurture others while abstaining oneself are all ultimately sought in and of themselves. For both the medieval "holy" anorexic back then and the individual with anorexia nervosa today, the self-sacrifice and other behaviors and compulsive devotion that are initially rewarded and praised become self-destructive and life threatening.

Richard Morton in London made the first formal description of anorexia nervosa in medical literature in 1689, which described both radical wasting and a loss of appetite that did not seem to be caused by medical symptoms but rather by sadness and anxiety. Morton is known for his description of a patient as "a skeleton clad only with skin." Two other physicians, Charles Lasegue in 1873 in France and Sir William Gull in 1874 in England, wrote the first two articles about anorexia nervosa in modern medical literature and described the features still recognized today as being associated with this disorder. Gull came up with the term anorexia nervosa to distinguish the disorder as being caused by a "morbid mental state" rather than a physiological cause.

Binge eating, which most people consider a third eating disorder, seems to have been around for centuries but was probably not recognized as a separate eating disorder because of the overlap with obesity. Obesity is understood as a medical illness, and thus the identification of a subgroup of obese or overweight individuals who also have the psychiatric component of binge eating may have been thwarted. It was not until 1990 that researchers recognized a binge eating syndrome that was not synonymous with bulimia nervosa or obesity, and in fact people who had it could be a normal weight. In 1994 BED was officially designated as a criteria set in need of further study in the *DSM-IV-TR*.

Eating disorders have been poorly understood for most of their history. Not until the 1930s did researchers believe the causes of self-starvation were psychological and emotional. To read more about the history of eating disorders, readers are referred to Joan Brumberg's *Fasting Girls: The History of Anorexia Nervosa* (1989) and Richard Gordon's *Eating Disorders: Anatomy of a Social Epidemic* (2000). Today, eating disorders are best understood as a combination of emotional factors interacting with biological and physiological imbalances (including the imbalances caused by dieting) in a vulnerable individual living in a cultural climate that places an emphasis on external appearance and thinness.

10. When does disordered eating become an eating disorder?

Many people are on diets, are concerned about their appearance, or have lost weight, tried laxatives, or occasionally binged. To know when someone has gone from a diet to a disorder, it is important to understand the clinical diagnostic criteria for each of the eating disorders listed in Question 1 above. It is also important to understand that crossing over into a disorder does not happen overnight, so any signs of food restriction, compulsive dieting, food rituals, lying about food, and so on, should be carefully monitored. A person should be in control of a diet, not have the diet control him or her. In eating disorders the person no longer seems to have control or a choice about his or her behaviors but rather is controlled by the rules of the "diet." People with eating disorders lie, hide, sneak, steal, give up social activities, put other things and other people off, beg when they believe their behaviors will not be allowed, deny when confronted with the reality of their situation even in the face of evidence, and even make threats to those trying to "interfere" or help.

11. Is it true that exercise can be a form of purging?

Exercise is a good thing, but many individuals use it as a way to burn off unwanted calories.

Exercise is a good thing, but many individuals use it as a way to burn off unwanted calories. Unfortunately, this can turn into a method of trying to burn off any calories consumed to the point where the individual believes he or she cannot eat without exercising. Compulsively exercising is often associated with eating disorders. At one point, exercise was considered a form of "purging," but now it is listed in the *DSM-IV-TR* criteria for bulimia nervosa as a "nonpurging" compensatory behavior, used to avoid weight gain or accomplish weight loss. See Question 12 for more information.

12. My therapist says I am a compulsive exerciser, but I say exercise is healthy. Who is right?

Like a diet that turns into an eating disorder, exercise can turn into a disorder too. Some individuals no longer choose to exercise but are driven to do it. These people often feel horrible about themselves when they do not exercise, give up social activities to exercise, cannot take rest days, and cannot stop even when exhausted or injured. Anyone with these symptoms has a problem and should try to get help. Exercising one's body is a good healthy thing to do, but when taken too far it is detrimental not only for the body, but for the mind. You do not need to have an eating disorder to be a compulsive exerciser, but many people who have eating disorders also have problems with compulsive exercise. Therefore professionals with expertise in eating disorders are the best to consult when someone has this problem.

People with anorexia and bulimia often have high levels of anxiety, obsessive-compulsive behaviors, and perfectionism, and it makes sense that they would be driven to use as many behaviors as possible to control weight. Professionals in the field have long noted that excessive exercise is a common feature of anorexia and bulimia, but it has been unclear which type of individual is most likely to have the problem.

To determine the type of female more likely to engage in excessive exercise, Dr. Cynthia M. Bulik and a team of researchers from Chapel Hill North Carolina looked at data from three international studies of women with anorexia, bulimia, or both. The women were asked questions on eating disorder symptoms, personality traits, and exercise habits. For the study excessive exercise was defined as exercising more than 3 hours a day or being so obsessed with daily physical activity that it interfered with other aspects of life, such as exercising even when injured or ill.

The study found that excessive exercise was common in women with anorexia and bulimia but most common among individuals with anorexia who purged. Of the 336 women in the study, more than half exercised excessively. However, it is important for professionals to look for symptoms of compulsive exercise in all their clients. If compulsive exercise is not treated, this feature presents a high risk for relapse.

If you have symptoms of compulsive exercise, you should get help. You can learn how to put exercise in its proper perspective for a healthy and balanced life.

13. My daughter is an athlete and I have heard that many athletes have eating disorders. How can I protect her?

It is a good idea to be concerned about any female in competitive sports, especially sports that tend to place an emphasis on the athlete's appearance and size. Many of these athletes have coaches who push weight loss, and some sports, like wrestling, even have weight requirements. A study of Division 1 National Collegiate Athletic Association athletes revealed that over one-third of female athletes reported attitudes and symptoms placing them at risk for anorexia nervosa. As is true for the general population, most athletes with eating disorders are female, but male athletes are also at risk.

If your daughter is an athlete, one particular thing to be aware of is a condition referred to as "the female athlete triad," which includes (1) disordered eating, (2) loss of menstrual periods, and (3) **osteoporosis**. This is a very serious condition because the lack of nutrition resulting from disordered eating can cause a change in hormone levels and the loss of several or more consecutive periods. For a long time the lack of menstruation was considered such a common occurrence among female athletes that no one took it too seriously. Now we know that this condition leads to calcium and bone loss, putting the athlete at greatly increased risk for stress fractures of the bones. Separately, disordered eating, loss of menstruation,

Osteoporosis

A disease of the bones in which the bone mineral density is reduced.

and osteoporosis are all serious concerns, but together they create serious health risks that are irreversible and possibly life threatening. Adolescent girls are most at risk for the female athlete triad because of the active biological changes and growth spurts they go through at this time; the insecurities that go along with adolescence, including peer and social pressures; and the increased focus on thinness for females. Males, however, may develop similar syndromes. The International Olympic Committee recognized this problem and continues to try to address this issue. There is now a handbook, *NCAA Coaches Handbook: Managing the Female Athlete Triad*, which should be consulted regarding this issue.

The following list gives risk factors that can contribute to an athlete developing an eating disorder. If you are a parent you can watch for these:

- Sports that emphasize appearance or weight requirements (e.g., gymnastics, diving, body building, or wrestling, i.e., wrestlers trying to "make weight").
- Sports that focus on the individual rather than the entire team (e.g., gymnastics, running, figure skating, dance, or diving).
- Endurance sports (e.g., track and field/running, swimming).
- Inaccurate belief that lower body weight improves performance.
- Training for a sport since childhood or being an elite athlete.
- Low self-esteem; family dysfunction; families with eating disorders; chronic dieting; history of physical or sexual abuse; peer, family, and cultural pressures to be thin; and other traumatic life experiences.

- Coaches who focus only on success and performance rather than on the athlete as a whole person.

It is important to note that the characteristics of someone with anorexia (i.e., perfectionism, tenacity, overlooking pain, mind over matter, self-sacrificing) are all qualities coaches consider attributes and thus look for in an athlete. This makes it more difficult to identify athletes who have eating disorders or are at risk for developing an eating disorder. Furthermore, coaches and loved ones should be particularly careful of overly praising these qualities. Ron Thompson and Brenda Sherman discuss this issue in their article, "'Good athlete' traits and characteristics of anorexia nervosa: Are they similar?", in *Eating Disorders, The Journal of Treatment and Prevention* (1999).

The following are protective factors for any parent, loved one, or professional to consider:

- It is important to pay attention to the athlete's focus on appearance and weight. Be proactive if you see any weight loss. Make sure you dispel the myth that performance is always improved by greater thinness.

- If you can, try to find coaches that pay specific attention to their athlete's health. Coaches should care more about their athlete than they do about performance. Coaches can have a profound influence and can be the first to notice problems if they pay attention.

- Athletes are usually quite driven on their own. A positive approach and coaching style is far better than criticism and negative reinforcement, which can drive athletes to ignore physical symptoms and to not care about themselves.

- Look for a team in which there is a healthy supportive atmosphere toward size and shape. Avoid coaches who emphasize body weight or shape, criticize their athletes for this, post these figures, or even shame athletes.

- Provide good education for athletes on adequate nutrition and consequences of improper eating in the long run.

- Although this is difficult to do, if the athlete continues to eat improperly, lose weight, or does not menstruate, limit sports participation and possibly pull him or her off the sport until he or she gets better.

14. How common are eating disorders?

It is unclear how many people suffer from eating disorders. Researchers have tried to do surveys in the community and in treatment programs to ascertain the prevalence of eating disorders, but the results are confusing. Many cases go unreported, and research is carried out in many different ways, making it hard to tell how many people actually have these disorders. Also, age groups vary in terms of prevalence of the illness. It is clear that anorexia nervosa is the rarest of all the eating disorders, but roughly 90% of those who get anorexia are adolescent females. If you check websites, books, and articles on eating disorders you will find a variety of figures on the estimated prevalence of these illnesses. The truth is we are not sure; consider these statements from various books and websites on eating disorders:

- The number of people with eating disorders and borderline conditions is three times the number of people living with AIDS in the United States.

- Up to 2% of adults in the United States have BED.
- Five to 10 million people in the United States suffer from eating disorders.
- One percent of female adolescents have anorexia and 4% of college women have bulimia.
- Five to 10 million young girls and 1 million boys and men are struggling with eating disorders.

Depending on where you look, you will find different answers to the question of how common eating disorders are. There are several sources and websites, such as The Eating Disorders Coalition (see Resources for more details), that provide the same overview of lifetime prevalence. These figures seem the most useful because they are listed as ranges rather than as static numbers. These sites all report that from 0.5% to 3.7% of females suffer from anorexia, and, as all clinicians and researchers agree, there are far more individuals who suffer from bulimia, at about 1.1% to 4.2%. The Eating Disorders Coalition site lists the prevalence of BED at 2% to 5% of males and females. It seems obvious that EDNOS would have far more numbers even still. However, EDNOS has not been sufficiently studied, and it is difficult to ascertain the prevalence rate at the present time. In fact, most of the discussions regarding prevalence rates of eating disorders refer to anorexia and bulimia, and only lately has BED been included.

15. Are eating disorders an adolescent illness?

The one thing we do know from research is that most people suffering from an eating disorder are female adolescents. However, eating disorders affect all ages. Eating disorder professionals and treatment programs are increasingly seeing both younger and older clients coming for treatment. In 2006 one representative of a residential eating disorder program reported that admissions of women over 40 have increased 400%. Younger children with eating disorders is also a growing problem, not just in this country but in others as well. Experts in Australia have also expressed concern over the number of children being hospitalized with eating disorders, which has tripled in the past 2 years, with sufferers as young as 10 being admitted with anorexia and bulimia.

Many professionals in the field say society's obsession with rising obesity, which has led to things like body fat report cards in schools, has caused 4-year-olds and 5-year-olds to worry about getting fat, with an alarming rise of admissions of young children to hospitals who have signs and symptoms of anorexia and bulimia. Of particular concern is the increase in admissions of those under age 14, which reportedly rose from 5 in 2003 to 25 in 2005, according to a study published in the *International Journal of Eating Disorders* in September 2006.

16. Do males really get eating disorders?

Eating disorders are not just a female issue. Several sources report that about 5% to 10% of individuals who suffer from anorexia or bulimia are males (Gordon, 2000; Keel, 2005). In their book on males with eating and body image problems, *Making Weight: Men's Conflicts with Food, Weight, Shape and Appearance* (2000), Andersen, Cohn, and Holbrook report Canadian studies that found that one in six cases of anorexia or bulimia are in men and that BED is almost equally present in men and women. These authors believe that males with eating disorders could represent as many as 25% to 30% of all cases, but they are underdiagnosed. Men are not as likely to seek treatment for an eating disorder, and clinicians are less likely to

Eating disorders are not just a female issue.

diagnose a male with an eating disorder. Furthermore, diagnostic criteria that existed for a number of years, like amenorrhea for anorexia, excluded males.

17. Do other ethnic groups get eating disorders?

Contrary to what was commonly thought and portrayed in the media, eating disorders exist in all kinds of ethnic groups. It does appear that those who seek and receive treatment for an eating disorder are more likely to be white females, and this has perpetuated a tendency to believing that they were more likely to develop eating disorders. For a more thorough discussion of this topic, readers can refer to Pamela Keel's book, *Eating Disorders* (2003). In summary, Keel says, "With the exception of African American or black women, most women of color appear to have the same risk of developing eating disorders as white women." It seems that black females do develop eating disorders but at a lower rate than white females; this is especially true for anorexia nervosa.

18. Are there eating disorders in other countries?

Eating disorders are now occurring everywhere. We have known for a while about their prevalence in countries considered more Westernized than others, such as Europe and many Latin American countries, for example, Argentina or Brazil. But we are increasingly seeing eating disorders in other countries, such as China, India, Japan, Africa, and Hong Kong. It appears that the more Westernized a country becomes, the more eating disorders become prevalent. Studies have also demonstrated that if individuals of various ethnic groups move to a more Westernized area, they develop more eating disorders. This issue is discussed in *Body Wars: Making Peace With Women's Bodies—An Activist's Guide* by Margo Maine and *The Body Myth: Adult Women and the Pressure to Be Perfect* by Margo Maine and Joe Kelly.

19. I have heard that people with eating disorders often have other problems and diagnoses. What are they?

Often, but not always, individuals who have eating disorders have other symptoms and problems that are not part of the diagnostic criteria for their eating disorder. It is not uncommon to see in bulimia and anorexia symptoms such as self-cutting or other self-harming behaviors that also need to be a focus of treatment.

Individuals with anorexia and bulimia may also suffer from some kind of anxiety disorder, depressive or other mood disorder, **body dysmorphic disorder**, and personality disorder (such as borderline personality disorder). People with anorexia are more likely to have obsessive-compulsive disorder (OCD) or social phobia, whereas people with bulimia or anorexia, binge/purge type, are more likely to also have substance abuse disorders.

For an additional diagnosis, it is important that these other illnesses present their symptoms in areas other than food and weight issues; otherwise, the symptoms might just be a part of the eating disorder. For example, if someone has true OCD, he or she exhibits obsessions and compulsions related to things like checking doors or hand washing in addition to those related to food and weight. If the individual has true body dysmorphic disorder, then the imagined defect in bodily appearance, characteristic of this disorder, shows up in other areas. I once saw a young man with anorexia nervosa and body dysmorphic disorder who not only obsessed about calories and weight but also about several body image

Body dysmorphic disorder

A preoccupation with an imagined physical defect in appearance or a vastly exaggerated concern about a minimal defect.

issues, including hatred for his freckles, which he saw as defects. This young man would not go out in sunlight unless fully covered, including gloves, for fear of getting freckles. He once tried to erase his freckles with a pencil eraser to the point of producing burns on his skin.

20. My wife has an eating disorder but she is also depressed. Will her eating disorder go away if the depression is treated?

It is not uncommon for people with eating disorders to have depression or at least depressive symptoms, but it is often unclear if one or the other came first. Most often, but not always, depression begins at the same time as bulimia. If it is known that a person suffering from an eating disorder in fact did have depression before the eating disorder, then treatment for depression, including medication, may help resolve the depression and the eating disorder. In any case, nutritional rehabilitation is a necessary first step because this alone can help alleviate symptoms of depression and is also usually necessary for medication to work, especially in the case of underweight individuals.

21. My daughter has bulimia and is also addicted to cocaine. Are they related and which should be treated first?

About 30% of those with bulimia also have a substance abuse problem, usually with alcohol or stimulants. Stimulant use, especially among females, often begins as a weight control method but becomes much more to the individual. Daily use presents a variety of problems such as inability to sleep, anxiety, paranoia, and overall loss of ability to function normally. Some people require chemical dependency treatment along with treatment for the eating disorder. Unless an individual needs to detox first, I believe it is a mistake to send someone to chemical dependency treatment first, believing the eating disorder can be dealt with later. This prolongs treatment and often postpones dealing with the motivation for the substance use. Individuals who have both problems, whether it involves alcohol or drugs, need a good program that can deal with both issues simultaneously because they are intertwined.

22. My daughter has always been very anxious and now she has lost a lot of weight. My wife believes she has an eating disorder, but I believe it is her anxiety. What should we do?

A history of anxiety is common in individuals who develop anorexia and bulimia. Your daughter could have an anxiety disorder and an eating disorder. On the other hand, appetite and weight loss can occur from anxiety without resulting in an eating disorder. Determining whether she also has a preoccupation with her weight and shape will help to determine whether she has an eating disorder, even if she does not meet the full criteria. In any case, before the problem goes too far you should consult an eating disorder professional who can assess the situation and advise you. It is important not to let your daughter be the guide here. Too often parents make the mistake of believing their daughter or son can turn things around. Often, the child does not believe he or she has an eating disorder and resists going anywhere to get help. Even if they know they have an eating problem, young people are very likely to resist any attempts to get help. Parents have to be together and be strong. Eating disorders are serious illnesses and should be treated as soon as possible. If parents suspect that their daughter or son has an eating disorder, they should act on it immediately. Not much harm is done if the parents are wrong, but a great deal of harm is likely to ensue if they are right and do not act.

23. I have obsessive-compulsive disorder. Does this mean I don't really have anorexia?

Having OCD or any other disorder does not mean you do not have an eating disorder. If you meet the criteria for an eating disorder and you have other obsessive-compulsive symptoms, you need to get help for both disorders. It is often hard to tell whether a person with anorexia has OCD or whether the starvation has caused obsessive and compulsive symptoms. Often, people with anorexia have various symptoms similar to someone with OCD. Usually, the symptoms are based around food, eating rituals, and weight, but often there are other OCD symptoms as well. For most of these people, weight gain and nutritional rehabilitation resolves or at least mitigates the OCD symptoms. If the person has true OCD and anorexia, it is often noted that OCD symptoms occurred before the eating disorder diagnosis. For example, before the eating disorder the person had hand-washing behaviors or checking behaviors, such as checking all the doors to make sure they were locked over and over again. If these kinds of behaviors were present before the eating disorder and persist after, then treatment for OCD is necessary as well. It is not always clear whether true OCD exists, but sometimes it is clear from the person's history that true OCD and an eating disorder are present and can both be treated at the same time.

24. I have heard about Pro-ana websites. What are these?

Pro-ana (anorexia) and Pro-mia (bulimia) websites promote eating disorders as life-style choices, not illnesses. Typical information found on these websites is as follows:

> "Welcome to a community of people who live with an eating disorder and want a chance to meet others in the same position, and talk without fear of judgment. Any type of person with any type of eating disorder is welcomed with open arms, it is a place to get support. THIS IS A PRO ED COMMUNITY. If it offends anyone, simply do not join or post.

> "We as ana pride, do not want to be normal, we do not want to get fat again, we want to be skinny and perfect, forever, and that is why we are ana. I am ana pride and wear a red yarn bracelet (the national symbol for ana pride) on my left wrist."

It is unclear who runs these sites and what their true motivation is, but they are detrimental in that they advocate strategies for how to better achieve success at getting and staying thin. Among other things, these sites post photos of very sick emaciated individuals, including celebrities, referring to them as "thinspiration."

Typical information found on these websites is as follows:

> Wearing red or other colorful armbands may be a symbol of involvement with these sites. If someone is on these sites, it might interfere with seeking and or getting help. If you know people visiting these sites, it is important to talk to them about their interest in the sites and help them to feel understood, without their having to resort to visiting these sites.

PART TWO

Medical Issues Associated with Eating Disorders

What is the role of the physician in the treatment of an eating disorder?

What are the medical complications involved in eating disorders?

What medical tests should I have done if I have an eating disorder?

More...

25. What is the role of the physician in the treatment of an eating disorder?

A physician is a critical part of a good treatment team. The physician needs to rule out any medical causes to help with proper diagnosis and treatment. For example, a young girl was referred to me with the idea that she had anorexia. A medical examination revealed she had severe gastric reflux and a hiatal hernia, causing her food refusal. She did not have an eating disorder but had several eating disorder–like symptoms. The physician needs to perform a complete medical examination on individuals suspected of having an eating disorder and should also be involved in continued medical monitoring. These illnesses are dangerous, and there are a variety of medical complications associated with them, some of which can be fatal. Be aware that it might be difficult for a physician to determine whether an individual has an eating disorder or not. People with eating disorders often do not tell the truth about their behaviors, and normal laboratory results are not an indication of an absence of an eating disorder. People can lose weight, vomit, take laxatives, and excessively exercise and still have laboratory results in normal ranges. In fact, by the time things show up on medical tests, there might be quite a bit of damage and an entrenched disorder. Sometimes it is important to get baseline values to use against tests taken further down the road. For example, a thyroid test or bone density test that is normal now may show up as low normal or abnormal down the road.

In addition, physicians are also called on to support the rest of the treatment team and are key participants in making decisions regarding treatment, such as whether or not to hospitalize an individual or allow them to participate in sports. Often, because of a lack of resources or because he or she is the most appropriate for the task, physicians are asked to weigh patients and monitor their weight and even deal with nutritional issues. Finally, some medical doctors who are not psychiatrists prescribe **psychotropic** medications for their patients with eating disorders. This usually happens when there are no other resources for the patient to get these medicines.

> **Psychotropic**
>
> A drug capable of affecting the mind; for example, one used to treat psychiatric disorders.

26. What are the medical complications involved in eating disorders?

The medical complications for eating disorders are quite varied. Different people get different symptoms. Some problems are caused by starvation or malnutrition, and others are caused from purging methods such as laxative abuse or vomiting. A variety of medical problems occur as a result of excessive weight gain from binging. Refer to the following alphabetical list for the various medical complications usually seen in eating disorder clients.

- *Acid reflux:* This is very common in eating disorders, especially in people with bulimia. The valve that should control stomach acid becomes faulty. Partially digested items in the stomach, mixed with acid and enzymes, leak back into the esophagus and even the mouth. Reflux can sometimes become severe enough that food cannot be kept down at all, and medical attention should be sought immediately. Persistent unremitting reflux can cause a serious condition called Barrett's esophagus, which is a change in the cells within the esophagus that can lead to cancer.

- *Amenorrhea* (loss of the menstrual cycle): Lack of adequate nutrition results in insufficient hormone levels and often, but not always, weight loss and loss of body fat. Some combination of these factors causes the loss of menstruation, and a loss of bone density (discussed next).

- *Bone density problems*: Thinning of the bones is one of the most serious and possibly irreversible problems with eating disorders, especially in anorexia nervosa. Individuals who have amenorrhea over a period of time lose bone density and can end up with osteopenia, which is below-normal bone mass, or osteoporosis, where the bone loss has become sufficient enough to be called a disease. In osteoporosis the reduction in bone mass causes the bones to be porous and to fracture or break easily.

- *Bruising of the skin*: Low blood pressure, low platelet count, extreme weight loss, and vitamin/mineral deficiencies all lead to easily bruised skin that can take a long time to heal.

- *Cardiovascular* (slowed or irregular heartbeat, arrhythmias, angina, heart attack): Many factors associated with eating disorders can lead to heart problems or a heart attack. Sudden cardiac arrest is one of the leading causes of death in anorexia nervosa, and there is speculation that this is true for bulimia also. Electrolyte imbalances (especially potassium deficiency), dehydration, low blood pressure, extreme **orthostatic hypotension**, and abnormally slow heart rate all can cause serious problems with the heart. Excessive weight can cause high blood pressure, accumulation of fat deposits around the heart muscle, high cholesterol, and hormonal imbalances, which also lead to serious problems with the heart.

- *Dehydration*: This can be caused by depleting the body of fluids by vomiting, laxative or diuretic abuse, or by the lack of intake of sufficient fluids. It is interesting to note that dehydration can also

Orthostatic hypotension

A sudden fall in blood pressure that occurs when a person assumes a standing position.

be caused by restriction of carbohydrates and fat. Symptoms include dizziness, weakness, or darkening of urine and can lead to kidney failure, heart failure, seizures, brain damage, and death.

- *Dental problems*: Stomach acids from vomiting cause erosion of tooth enamel, severe decay, and gum disease. Vitamin D, calcium deficiencies, and hormonal imbalance cause decalcification of the teeth.

- *Digestive difficulties:* A deficiency in digestive enzymes leads to the body's inability to properly digest food and absorb nutrients. This can lead to malabsorption problems, malnutrition, and electrolyte imbalances. Delayed gastric emptying is common, and individuals complain of early **satiety**. Digestive enzymes and/or a medication to speed gastric emptying may be necessary.

- *Dry skin, hair, and nails and hair loss:* This is caused by vitamin and mineral deficiencies, malnutrition, and dehydration.

- *Edema*: Swelling of the soft tissues is the result of excess water accumulation from laxative or diuretic abuse. This may also been seen in refeeding edema (see Question 32).

- *Electrolyte Imbalances*: Electrolytes are essential to the production of the body's natural impulses to the nerves, muscles, and organs and to the delivery of oxygen to the cells. Eating disorder patients can die from cardiac arrest due to electrolyte imbalance. Low potassium (hypokalemia) and high bicarbonate (metabolic alkalosis) are the most common electrolyte abnormalities seen in patients who purge either with diuretics or

Satiety

From the Latin *satietas*, from *satis*, "enough." Refers to the psychological feelings of "fullness" or satisfaction rather than to the physical feeling of being engorged (i.e., the feeling of physical fullness after eating a very large meal).

with vomiting; these abnormalities are potentially the most dangerous. Hypokalemia can cause cardiac conduction defects, and arrhythmias and metabolic alkalosis can cause seizures and arrhythmias. Laxative abuse often, but not always, causes a low potassium level, a low bicarbonate level, and a high chloride level, together referred to as hyperchloremic metabolic acidosis.

- *Gastrointestinal complaints* (cramps, bloating, constipation, diarrhea, and incontinence): Bowel and stomach complaints are the most common. There can be increased or decreased bowel activity. Lack of food or cessation of laxative use may lead to severe constipation, and if there is pain and the constipation persists, a blockage should be ruled out. Gastric rupture has occurred from binging, and sometimes there is gastrointestinal bleeding into the digestive tract.

- *Hypo- and Hyperglycemia*: Hypoglycemia (low blood sugar) can indicate problems with the liver or kidneys and can lead to neurological and mental deterioration. Hyperglycemia (high blood sugar as a result of low production of insulin) can be a result of poor eating habits and excess weight and can lead to diabetes.

- *Hyponatremia* (low sodium): Water is good for us, but eating disorder clients often drink too much, believing it is healthy, using it to distract from hunger, or "water loading" to artificially raise their scale weight for a weigh in. Drinking too much water (more than eight 8-ounce glasses in less than 12 hours) can cause fluid in the lungs, the brain to swell, nauseousness, vomiting, confusion, and even death.

- *Infertility*: Loss of menstrual cycle, hormonal imbalances, malnutrition, and vitamin deficiencies can affect the ability to have children and can also increase problems with pregnancy and birth defects. Additionally, at least one study has suggested that people with eating disorders were at an increased risk for developing **polycystic ovarian syndrome**.

- *Iron-deficiency anemia*: Low iron makes the oxygen-transporting units within the blood useless and can lead to fatigue, shortness of breath, increased infections, and heart palpitations.

- *Ketoacidosis*: A high level of acids build up in the blood (known as ketones) when the body burns fat instead of sugar and carbohydrate. This can lead to coma and death. This problem has arisen with people on high fat and severely low carbohydrate diets, such as the Atkins diet. Ketoacidosis can be caused by starvation, excessive purging, dehydration, hyperglycemia, alcohol abuse, and diabetes.

- *Kidney infection and failure*: Kidneys are the body's clearinghouse. Our kidneys clear poisons from the body, regulate acid concentration, and maintain water balance. Dehydration, infection, and low blood pressure increase the risks of kidney problems.

- *Lanugo* (soft downy hair on face, back, and arms): There is a protective mechanism built into our bodies to help keep us warm during periods of starvation and malnutrition. This mechanism causes us to grow fine hair on the body to protect it from the cold. Occasionally, the eyelashes of a person with an eating disorder get fuller as part of this same mechanism.

Polycystic ovarian syndrome

Characterized by changes to the ovaries such that multiple follicles accumulate in the ovaries without ovulation.

- *Liver failure*: The liver aids in removing waste from cells and aids in digestion. Loss of menstruation, dehydration, and chronic heart failure can lead to liver damage or failure.

- *Low blood pressure or hypotension*: Low blood pressure can be caused by starvation, lowered body temperature, malnutrition, and dehydration. This can cause heart arrhythmias, shock, or cardiac arrest. Orthostatic hypotension occurs when there is a sudden drop in blood pressure upon sitting up or standing. Symptoms include dizziness, blurred vision, fainting, heart pounding, and headaches.

- *Low body temperature*: Most people with anorexia and some with bulimia complain of being cold all the time. This is caused by low blood pressure and the loss of body fat and muscle. The healthy insulating layer of fat that normally protects from the cold is gone and the person is not eating enough to generate heat.

- *Low platelet count*: This is caused by low levels of vitamin B12 and folic acid and/or by excessive alcohol use. It may also be an indication of a suppressed or deficient immune system.

- *Malnutrition*: Malnutrition means there is a deficiency in some or all of the following: calories, protein, fat, carbohydrates, certain nutrients, or micronutrients necessary for health. Malnutrition can cause severe health risks, including (but not limited to) respiratory infections, kidney failure, blindness, heart attack, and death.

- *Muscle atrophy*: Lack of nutrition and calories causes muscle wasting as the body feeds off of itself. Impaired neuromuscular functioning can develop from vitamin and mineral deficiencies, especially potassium. Some clients even experience temporary paralysis where they have extreme weakness of muscles and find it difficult or impossible to move. I have seen clients unable to walk as if their legs were made of rubber. This can result from low levels of potassium and/or the degeneration of nerve cells in the spinal cord or in the brain, which have been deprived of essential nutrients. Left untreated, temporary paralysis may become more frequent and severe, leading to permanent muscle weakness and even death.

- *Pancreatitis*: Excessive use of laxatives or diet pills can cause digestive enzymes to attack the pancreas, causing pancreatitis.

- *Parotid gland swelling*: Parotid glands (salivary glands) are located behind the cheek and under the ear. Both parotid glands swell as a result of vomiting, usually after an individual has stopped for a day or more. The swelling makes the person look like they have the mumps. To help alleviate the swelling, the person can suck on tart candies.

- *Seizures*: There seems to be an increased risk of seizures in individuals with anorexia and bulimia, which may be caused by dehydration, hyperglycemia, or ketoacidosis. It is also possible that long-term malnutrition and lack of oxygen-carrying cells to the brain may play a role.

- *Sleep problems*: Eating disorder clients often have problems falling and/or staying asleep, which could be caused by a variety of issues.

- *Tearing of esophagus*: Tiny tears, known as Mallory-Weiss tears, can be caused by repeated forceful self-induced vomiting. Individuals may notice blood in their vomit, but this condition is not usually dangerous.
- *Weakness and fatigue*: This is caused by generalized poor eating habits, electrolyte imbalances, vitamin and mineral deficiencies, depression, malnutrition, and heart problems.

Some medical consequences are not too serious, and most reverse with nutritional rehabilitation and recovery. However, it is important to remember that death can be caused by a variety of medical complications arising from eating disorders, and these should always be under scrutiny: heart failure, lung collapse, internal bleeding, stroke, kidney failure, seizure, liver failure, pancreatitis, gastric rupture, and suicide.

27. What medical tests should I have done if I have an eating disorder?

It is important for the physician not only to check for any existing medical issues or complications that must be attended to but also to establish a baseline for future comparisons. For example, a person's thyroid or bone density test taken several months apart may indicate results in the normal range but at the same time show a trend downward, which would be important information. A brief summary of medical tests taken in eating disorder patients is listed here. Other books, such as *The Eating Disorder Sourcebook* (Costin, 2007), provide more detailed information for readers on medical tests and issues.

Vital signs such as temperature, heart rate, and blood pressure should all be taken along with weight (See more about weight in Part Four.) and monitored throughout treatment as necessary. Low body temperature and pulse rates that are either too low (**bradycardia**) or too high (**tachycardia**) should be investigated and monitored closely. Blood pressure changes, for example, from sitting to standing, may be dangerous and the person might need to be referred to a hospital or treatment program.

Bradycardia

A pulse rate that is too low. Slowness of the heart rate is usually measured as fewer than 60 beats/minute in an adult human.

It is important for a physician to order an "eating disorder laboratory panel" as part of the medical assessment. This panel of tests may include those not routinely performed in a physical examination but that should be done with an eating disordered patient. The following laboratory tests are generally recommended:

Tachycardia

A pulse rate that is too high; an excessively rapid heartbeat, typically regarded as a heart rate exceeding 100 beats/minute in a resting adult.

- Complete blood count. (CBC).
- Chem-20 panel: Measures electrolytes, liver, kidney, and pancreatic function. Total protein and albumin, calcium, and sedimentation rates should be included.
- Sma-7 or electrolytes: This test is usually included in the previously mentioned Chem-20 but sometimes doctors order this test alone.
- Magnesium and phosphorous levels: These levels are not regularly tested, but in anorexia, particularly with refeeding, they should be tested and monitored.
- Serum amylase: Indicates pancreatic function and possibly purging.
- Thyroid and parathyroid panel: Indicates level of metabolic function.
- Hormone levels.

Other tests that are selectively performed are as follows:

- Electrocardiogram: (EKG) Measures heart function.

- Chest X-ray: Investigates chest pain.
- Abdominal X-ray: Investigates unremitting or painful constipation or stomach distension.
- Lower esophageal sphincter pressure studies for reflux: To investigate spontaneous vomiting or severe indigestion.
- Lactose deficiency tests for dairy intolerance: Investigates patient complaints and determines inability to digest dairy products.
- Total bowel transit time for severe constipation: Unremitting constipation accompanied by severe cramping and pain may indicate a blockage.
- C-3 complement level, serum ferritin, serum iron, and transferring saturation level: The most sensitive tests for protein and iron deficiency.
- Bone mineral density test: Numerous studies show that deficiency in bone mineral density (bone density) is a common and serious medical complication of eating disorders, particularly anorexia nervosa. Low levels of bone density can result in osteopenia or osteoporosis (discussed earlier in Question 26).
- Weight: A physician and/or someone else on the treatment team (often a nutritionist) needs to keep track of the patient's weight, to reassure the patient and to assess progress in treatment goals such as weight gain, when appropriate. The whole topic of weight needs more attention and is discussed further in Part Four, regarding seeing a nutritionist.

28. How do I know if I need a bone density test?

Bone density problems cannot be determined by cursory inspection but can be determined through testing. All clients who meet the criteria for anorexia nervosa as well as those with bulimia nervosa and a past episode of anorexia nervosa (up to 50% of persons with bulimia nervosa) should be tested. Other individuals who may not meet the full criteria for an eating disorder but who have had amenorrhea or intermittent menstrual periods may also need to be tested. There is increasing evidence that males with eating disorders are also likely to have bone density problems and therefore should be tested as well. For a sensitive and specific way to measure bone density, a **dual-energy X-ray absorptiometry (DEXA)** scan is recommended. This kind of scan is the most precise as it can measure small changes in bone mass and can be used to examine both the spine and extremities. Ask your doctor for this specific kind of bone density test.

DEXA
(Dual-energy x-ray absorptiometry scan) Currently, the most widely used method to measure bone mineral density.

29. My doctor says I have amenorrhea as a result of anorexia. Should I take hormone replacement therapy?

Hormone replacement therapy has not been established as a cure for, or prevention of, bone density problems in anorexia or bulimia. It appears that loss of bone density in anorexia is different from that in postmenopausal women and thus requires different treatment. It is also problematic to take hormone replacement therapy when trying to determine a healthy weight at which menstruation will resume normally. However, physicians often prescribe hormone replacement therapy for women who have suffered from amenorrhea because in some cases it seems to have helped and this is one of the only tools they have. It is now thought that hormone replacement therapy should not be prescribed unless amenorrhea has lasted for a long time (this depends on each case and each doctor, but a few months or even years may not warrant hormone replacement therapy). Other recommendations, such as taking 1,500 to 1,800 mg of calcium daily, are easy to do. New medications, such as Fosamax, are being tried for bone density problems but are still considered experimental. Ask a doctor trained in eating disorders what option is best for you.

30. I had amenorrhea but now I'm on the pill. Does this mean I don't have it anymore?

This line of thinking is dangerous. Taking the pill (hormone replacement therapy) is only a substitute for the real thing. It is a way scientists discovered to "fake" your body into having a period. You need to go off the pill to determine whether you are able to menstruate on your own. If an individual only menstruates due to replacement hormones, she still has amenorrhea.

31. My teeth are eroding. Is this from purging and is there anything I can do?

Purging (vomiting) erodes the enamel on the teeth from the stomach acid washing over the teeth. This causes loss of enamel, sensitivity, and cavities. Sometimes teeth erode from lack of nutrients as well, which is often seen in long-term anorexia nervosa.

32. What is refeeding syndrome

Refeeding syndrome occurs when starved or severely malnourished individuals undergo life-threatening fluid and electrolyte shifts after resuming a higher caloric intake. This syndrome can occur in patients on a pure

Refeeding syndrome

Occurs when previously malnourished patients are fed with high carbohydrate loads; the result is a rapid fall in phosphate, magnesium, and potassium.

food diet but is more common in those receiving either **enteral (tube feeding)** or **parenteral (intravenous feeding)** nutritional support. Refeeding syndrome is dangerous and can result in stress on the heart and even cardiac arrest. To avoid refeeding syndrome, electrolytes should be checked and normalized and calories should be increased slowly while ensuring adequate amounts of vitamins and minerals. Patients experience edema and a rapid pulse if they are developing refeeding syndrome; therefore these values should be frequently assessed and, if found, calories lowered immediately. Organ function, fluid balance, and serum electrolytes (especially phosphorus, potassium, and magnesium) need to be monitored several times a week in the beginning of refeeding and then less often thereafter, eventually returning to only routine checks.

Enteral
(Tube Feeding)

Literally means using the gastrointestinal tract for the delivery of nutrients, which includes eating food, consuming oral supplements, and all types of tube feeding.

Parenteral
(Intravenous Feeding)

Total parenteral nutrition is the practice of feeding a person intravenously, circumventing the gut.

33. I am pregnant and have an eating disorder. Will I hurt my baby?

Women with eating disorders have a higher risk of fertility problems, and those who get pregnant can be at a higher risk for miscarriage, high-risk pregnancy, and birth defects, including those that can cause the mother's or the baby's death. Women with anorexia nervosa may not gain enough weight during pregnancy and may have a baby with an abnormally low birth weight and related health problems. Women with bulimia nervosa or anyone who purges may suffer dehydration, chemical imbalances, or even cardiac irregularities, and pregnancy heightens these health risks. Women with binge eating disorder who are overweight are at greater risk of developing high blood pressure, gestational diabetes, and babies with abnormally high birth weights.

All medical issues associated with eating disorders could also affect a growing fetus. Risks can include:

- Miscarriage.
- Gestational diabetes.
- **Preeclampsia** (toxemia).
- Low amniotic fluid.
- Difficulties nursing.
- Premature birth.
- Placental separation.
- Complications during labor (such as a breech birth).
- Incompetent cervix.
- Delayed fetal growth.
- Low birth weight.
- Labor complications.
- Birth defects and fetal abnormality, such as a cleft palate.
- Respiratory distress of the baby immediately after birth.
- Postpartum depression.
- Higher possibility of death before or after birth
- **Low Apgar scores** (a reading of several features taken 1 and 5 minutes after birth: the baby's skin color, heart rate, movement, breathing, and reflexes, each rated from 0, poor, to 2, good).

Preeclampsia

A disorder that occurs only during pregnancy and the postpartum period and affects both the mother and the unborn baby.

Apgar score

A number arrived at by scoring the heart rate, respiratory effort, muscle tone, skin color, and response to a catheter in the nostril.

Of course, it is best to resolve any eating disorder–related weight and behavior problems before attempting to get pregnant. However, if you do become pregnant there is nothing more important than taking good care of yourself, which includes eating a well-balanced diet, drinking plenty of fluids, and taking prenatal vitamins or other supplements recommended by a physician. You should seek specialized medical help from a doctor who understands eating disorders and be sure you are getting psychological help as well. Remember that professionals can address the specific needs related to pregnancy and disordered eating only if you are willing to be completely honest with them.

The following list is a guide for those who have an eating disorder and wish to become pregnant or are currently pregnant and have an eating disorder:

- Find a physician who understands eating disorders long before becoming pregnant (if possible). You must be honest and tell the doctor your eating habits, fears, dieting practices and history, and any current eating disorder behaviors.

- Consult a nutritionist with expertise in eating disorders if possible before becoming pregnant. Work with the nutritionist and doctor throughout the pregnancy to get guidance on what and how much to eat and how to handle food fears. Stick with nutritional counseling for a while at least after you give birth in order to get expert and sensitive help to guide you through feelings about your weight and how to return to your normal weight in a healthy way.

- I recommend strongly that you ask your doctor or nutritionist (or both) to monitor your weight for you through this whole process because the number on the scale could potentially upset or trigger you. Stand on the scale backward and have the doctor or nutritionist keep the number private; he or she can offer advice and help you without your knowing a number and can tell you whether there is a problem in this area.

- You should be in therapy to help you overcome your eating disorder. You need help to cope with your concerns and fears regarding food, weight gain, body image, and all the feelings that go along with pregnancy, including your new role as a mother.

- Therapy sessions with your partner are also helpful. Your partner is in the best position to support you, but chances are you will need to work out his or her fears and concerns. Although each case is different, couples counseling can be done with your individual therapist.

- A prenatal exercise class and/or a support group for your eating disorder may be useful and help with physical and mental issues. Make sure your doctor and therapist are okay with whatever groups you wish to attend.

- Pregnancy, childbirth, child development, and parenting skills classes can also be helpful in preparing to become a mother.

- If you are taking medication for your eating disorder or related conditions, you need to consult with your doctor and psychiatrist to see whether you can continue to take them during this time.

34. I use laxatives to help me lose weight but now believe I am addicted. Does this mean I need to take them the rest of my life?

First, it is important to understand that laxatives are a very ineffective method to induce weight loss. Calories are absorbed in the small bowel, and laxatives affect the large bowel. What you do lose are large volumes of watery diarrhea and electrolytes. Usually, people with eating disorders are effectively weaned off laxatives even though it may take weeks to accomplish restoration of normal bowel habits. When coming off laxatives it is important to drink lots of fluids and eat a high-fiber diet. Exercise can also help but is not advised for severely underweight patients. Some individuals develop a laxative dependency, but this is not common. If constipation persists, a glycerin suppository, nonstimulating osmotic laxative, or a product called **MiraLax**, might be helpful but should be taken with the knowledge and approval of your doctor. In rare cases loss of colonic function can become so severe that a **colectomy** (surgery) is needed to treat intractable constipation. I treated a young woman of 26 and an older woman of 60 who both had so severely abused laxatives they had to be hooked up to a bag on a 24-hour basis because they had lost all ability to control their bowels.

MiraLax
A remedy for constipation.

Colectomy
Surgery during which all or part of the colon (also called the large intestine) is removed.

PART THREE

What Causes An Eating Disorder?

I often hear that eating disorders are all about control. Is this true?

Are eating disorders caused by the cultural emphasis on thinness?

Does the media cause eating disorders?

More...

35. I often hear that eating disorders are all about control. Is this true?

Believing that eating disorders are all about control is far too simplistic a view, but control issues do play a part. Clients themselves often talk about the issue of control and how it relates to their eating disorder. People who suffer from anorexia and bulimia can often be seen as trying to control something, and controlling their weight and food, what goes in and out of this body, is a metaphor for trying to control their life. People with binge eating disorder feel out of control with food. Helping people see how their relationship with food is like their relationship with people can help them learn things about the meaning of their symptoms. A person with anorexia might discover that she scrutinizes all food, everything she lets in, and she scrutinizes all people. She may be perfectionistic and fearful of food and people. Someone with bulimia might find that she binges and "purges" men. She may find herself getting into and out of several relationships. People with binge eating often describe feeling like they can never get enough food or enough out of relationships. They often fear being without either. I ask all my clients to write about how their relationship with food is like their relationship with people and go over this in therapy. Interventions can be made in either area that affects the other. You can help someone with their personal relationships and often their relationship to food gets better. Likewise, if you help them with their relationship with food, their personal relationships improve.

36. Are eating disorders caused by the cultural emphasis on thinness?

Over the last three decades I have heard story after story of young women trying to look like the latest super model, vomiting to lose weight for some event, taking laxatives to have a flat stomach on the beach, giving up everything for a number on the scale, and binging until too full and miserable to move because none of the other things worked out. I also suffered from my own eating disorder and felt first hand the pressure to diet, to get thin to be accepted, thinner to be admired, and the thinnest, to be exceptional and even envied. We live in a world where the cultural emphasis on appearance, and thinness specifically, is so common, so a part of the female vernacular, so much a part of what it means to be a female that it is hard to imagine a world without it. Caroline Knapp writes about this brilliantly in her book, *Appetites* (2003), "There is nothing new about this today; the pressure (internal and external) to be thin is so familiar and so widespread by now that most of us take it for granted, breathe it in like air, can't remember a time when we weren't aware of it, can't remember how different the average model or actress or beauty pageant contestant looked before her weight began to plummet (in the last twenty-five years it has dropped to twenty-five percent below that of the average woman), can't remember a world in which grocery store shelves didn't brim with low-cal and 'lite' products, in which mannequins wore size eight clothes instead of size two, in which images of beauty were less wildly out of reach."

The idea that losing weight will make us happy has led to a multibillion dollar industry, even though it is not true and dieting does not work, not in the long run anyway. However, we keep trying to make diets work in our pursuit to look like the images we see everywhere we turn. Supermodels, besides, weighing on average up to 25% less than their typical female counterparts in the "real" world, maintain a weight at about 15% to 20% below what is considered healthy for their age and height. Many look like they should be hospitalized for anorexia. In fact in the fall of 2006 one supermodel died right after coming off the modeling runway. This prompted a response from the organizers of Madrid fashion shows to send home all models under a BMI of 18 (which is considered to be a criteria for anorexia nervosa). The issue was fueled even more when soon after Brazilian model Ana Carolina Reston died from complications due to anorexia. In response to what became a worldwide focus on the issue of underweight models, the Council of Fashion Designers of America, led by president Diane von Furstenberg, issued a formal health initiative and guidelines in order to promote awareness, wellness, and a healthier work environment in the American fashion industry. It is unclear how the new guidelines will be enforced but this was a welcomed and long overdue reaction and response from the industry. It is the first step in the right direction. I hope to see much more of it.

Plastic surgery, liposuction, and airbrushing are commonly used to make models and actresses conform to the current ideal, and the public is following suit at an ever-increasing rate. Because these images and ideals are so pervasive in our culture, it is almost too difficult to determine the effects they have. Dieting is an accepted part of life, starving in order to fit into a certain size is part of being female, and a woman without a scale is hard to find.

In this climate, it is no wonder that females find dieting a solution not just for weight loss but also to gain status, power, control, and approval. Dieting and disordered eating can become a solution to other problems, and we know increased dieting leads to increased eating disorders. The cultural emphasis on female thinness is one of the only explanations so far that takes into account why eating disorders are an overwhelmingly female illness. But the words of Caroline Knapp are important to remember here, " Our culture's specific preoccupation with weight—particularly women's weight—has a lot to do with our more general preoccupation with women's bodies, not all of which is benign or caring, and a woman's individual preoccupation with weight often serves as a mask for other, more intricate sources of discomfort, the state of one's waistline being easier to contemplate than the state of one's soul."

Eating disorders are increasing in other cultures in a way that adds credence to the idea that the internalization of thinness is a significant contributing factor. The more modernized and Westernized a culture becomes, the more exposure to Western products, images, and ideas, the more eating disorders occur. This again points to the fact that, at least in part, Western culture's ideals of beauty, and particularly thinness, motivate eating disorder behaviors.

37. Does the media cause eating disorders?

The media is the way the culture gets disseminated, and we looked at the culture's effect on eating disorders in the previous question. More specifically, much evidence indicates that the media contributes to dieting, size discrimination, and body image dissatisfaction. These are all precursors of eating disorders. Research shows that as dieting articles in magazines increased over the years, so did eating disorders. The media contradicts the message that it is what's inside that counts and blatantly portrays that what you look like is more important than who you are. Thin women are idealized in every possible way, and fat people are made fun of. Images on television

Research shows that as dieting articles in magazines increased over the years, so did eating disorders.

show countless hours and advertisers spend countless dollars telling us to lose weight, be thin and beautiful, and that we need to buy and do the right things to make this happen.

The media obviously doesn't cause anorexia, bulimia, or binge eating; otherwise we would have a lot more cases than we see today. A variety of risk factors has to be in place for a full blown eating disorder to develop. These include psychological, genetic, biological, and cultural factors. However, the media promotes dieting and dieting is a risk factor. I would also go so far as to say that media images and advertising are probably responsible for a number of cases of what we referred to earlier in Part One as Eating Disorders Not Otherwise Specified. We have a society full of them.

With all the research that exists, the most interesting and compelling indictment of the media's role in eating disorders is what is known as the Fiji study. Anne Becker and colleagues at Harvard had the opportunity to investigate the effect of the introduction of television to the Fijian islands. Before 1995 Fijians did not watch television (because they did not have it), they did not diet, and there were no eating disorders. As I have heard Anne Becker describe it, in Fiji's 2000-year-old culture it was considered a bad thing to lose weight, and neighbors would come over to help fatten you up if you did. Starving or vomiting to lose weight was unthinkable, and eating disorders unheard of. In just 3 months after television was introduced, with Western programming like "Bay Watch," adolescent girls were engaged in dieting, and in 3 years time 11% were vomiting to lose weight! When asked, the Fijian girls reported among other things that they wanted to lose weight to increase their status. This is an astounding effect. Readers are encouraged to look up the study for more details (it is easy to find on the Internet). I believe the Fiji study is one of the most important pieces of research in the area of culture, the media, and eating disorders. Suffice it to say that if any drug or substance showed such dramatic negative effects, we would not let our children take it and we would stay as far away from it as we could get. Readers might want to consider this when deciding how much television watching to allow in the home. Additionally, it is wise to provide a wide variety of alternatives to television. Parents need to provide antidotes to the current bombardment children get of the wrong messages.

38. Do biological factors contribute to eating disorders?

Researchers are continually looking for any biological features that contribute to the development of eating disorders. So far no major breakthroughs have advanced our treatment strategies. Some initial investigations indicate that the **neurotransmitters** serotonin and dopamine might play a role in anorexia and bulimia, but researchers are unclear about exactly how this works and what can be done about it.

Neurotransmitters
Chemicals that are used to relay, amplify, and modulate electrical signals between a neuron and another cell.

Other biological abnormalities that may play a role in the development or perpetuation of eating disorders include:

- A defect in the endocrine system that affects appetite.
- A problem with stomach emptying such that the individual feels full longer.
- A problem with the body registering fullness or **satiety.**
- A deficiency in some vital nutrient such as zinc (see more about this in Part Ten).

At this point more research is necessary to confirm any biological contributions and to explore where this might lead in terms of treatment or prevention.

39. I heard eating disorders are genetic. Is this true?

There are a number of risk factors for developing an eating disorder, and it appears that genetics may be one of them. In the last few years researchers found new evidence regarding a genetic predisposition for developing an eating disorder. It first was discovered that eating disorders run in families. If a family member has an eating disorder, you have a greater chance of getting an eating disorder. The closer the relative, the greater the chance; therefore first-degree relatives (e.g., mother or sister) have the highest risk.

It is important to keep in mind that only about 5% to 10% of people with eating disorders have a close relative with an eating disorder.

It is important to keep in mind that only about 5% to 10% of people with eating disorders have a close relative with an eating disorder. We are not talking about a simple transmission of genes here. Research does indicate that genes may contribute in some way to the development of an eating disorder, but this is a very complex situation. The exact contribution of genes (probably several parts of several genes) and how this all gets transmitted is not understood. Family members, especially close ones, can also model behaviors, so it is unclear how much of the eating disorder behavior is learned. This is where the studies of twins are important.

Evidence shows us that identical twins get eating disorders at higher rates than fraternal (nonidentical) twins. Due to the fact that identical twins have the exact same genetic makeup, when they get a disorder at a higher rate than fraternal twins, genetics are thought to be the cause. However, some argue that these figures might be inflated and point out that identical twins share a more similar environment than fraternal twins and are treated more similarly and influence each other more than fraternal twins, all of which could be factors that cannot be separated out. In other words, if in fact identical twins share a more equal environment than fraternal twins, interpretation of the data toward genetics being responsible for greater eating disorders in identical twins may be skewed. To date, molecular studies, those that actually look for specific genes that increase the risk of developing an eating disorder, are very few and have yet to provide anything conclusive. Obviously more research is necessary.

Genetics do influence personality traits and temperament, including things that are thought to contribute to the development of an eating disorder, such as anxiety, compulsivity, or perfectionism. If 10 people go on a diet, it is perhaps the most compulsive and perfectionistic person who takes the dieting to an extreme and ends up with anorexia nervosa. It is quite plausible that genetic influences that determine temperament may be how genetics influence the development of an eating disorder.

40. My identical twin has anorexia. Will I automatically get it?

Having an identical twin with an eating disorder does not mean that you will automatically develop one. It does mean that, statistically, you have a greater chance of developing an eating disorder than a nontwin sibling. If a fraternal twin develops anorexia nervosa, her nonidentical twin gets it about 5% of the time. Researchers report that when an identical twin develops anorexia nervosa, the chances of her identical sister also getting it are around 56%. As previously mentioned in Question 39, it is not clear how much of this percentage jump is due to similar genetics or a more similar environment, but clearly identical twins are at a higher risk. The percentage of genetic contribution to the other eating disorders is even less clear.

Because there is evidence that identical twins are at a higher risk than normal, it would be wise to be alert to your own feelings about your body or tendencies to diet and to get help for yourself even if you do not have an eating disorder now. Talking about your feelings toward your twin and getting help on how to protect yourself from getting an eating disorder are important.

41. I had an eating disorder. What are the chances my daughter will develop one?

Eating disorders seem to run in families at a higher rate than in the general population, and first-degree relatives (mothers, sisters, daughters) of someone with an eating disorder have a greater chance of developing an eating disorder than other relatives. However, this by no means implies that if you have an eating disorder your daughter or any other relative will develop one; in fact, approximately 90% to 95% of the time they don't. Parents do not genetically transmit eating disorders to their kids. However, because she is statistically at a higher risk, it is important to be alert for any signs in your daughter and try to foster an environment that is an antidote to eating disorders. You should work actively to prevent an excessive focus on weight and appearance and encourage activities that are nonappearance focused. The best thing you can do for her is to be a good role model and take care of your own body. Dieting is a learned behavior. Healthy eating, exercise, and appearance-related behaviors and attitudes are important to model. Certainly the advice here applies to all parents, but because of the recent genetic findings, researchers emphasize this particularly for parents who have had or currently have eating disorders.

42. Do psychological problems cause eating disorders?

There are many reasons why people develop eating disorders. Many who suffer from these disorders also have depression or anxiety, which can cause or contribute to the eating disorder. Low self-esteem and self-esteem based on appearance seem to be contributing factors. Teasing and weight-related criticism by peers have been implicated in the drive for thinness and restrictive eating. There are all kinds of other psychological or personality problems that have been associated with eating disorders, including impulse control, affect regulation, perfectionism, obsessionality, and rejection sensitivity. None of these traits implies an eating disorder, but because people with eating disorders often have these traits, it is important to look for them. Eating disorder behaviors that started out as a means of dieting often become ways that a person with these traits learns to cope. For example, a highly rejection sensitive person can use weight loss as a way to try to gain acceptance and approval. A person lacking affect regulation and impulse control might try to diet but may be unable to follow a rigid diet plan. Upon breaking the diet this person might feel so bad she is driven to purge. Eventually, this same person, upon breaking her diet, might think, "Well I blew it anyway so I might as well eat everything I can since I am going to purge." This then becomes, "I am upset so I think I will go binge and purge." Eventually, the person has full-blown bulimia nervosa and is routinely engaging in the behaviors as a daily habit. Some people use binging to avoid feelings of emptiness. Some people with anorexia are so anxious that starving and being in such rigid control makes them feel safe and calm and it appears that this may have a biological component.

Over the last 30 years I have treated countless people with eating disorders and helped them learn how to utilize their traits to their advantage. It is a joy to watch someone turn her trait of perfectionism toward artistic talents or another more worthy goal than weight loss, to watch an anxious person learn to manage anxiety through yoga or meditation, or to watch someone who was badly mistreated or abused learn that it was not her fault and to not take it out on her body. Teaching people with eating disorders to deal positively with their temperament and to discover how their symptoms are helping them deal with other problems can be a key to helping them find other coping methods and thus help them fully recover.

43. I heard sexual abuse causes eating disorders. Is this true?

PTSD

(Posttraumatic stress disorder) A psychiatric disorder that can occur after the experience or witnessing of life-threatening events such as military combat, natural disasters, terrorist incidents, serious accidents, or violent personal assaults like rape.

Clinicians have long noticed that a subset of people who come for treatment for an eating disorder have a history of sexual abuse. It is clear that not everyone who has been sexually abused develops an eating disorder. For a long time the relationship between sexual abuse and eating disorders was unclear. The latest research shows that sexual abuse that results in **posttraumatic stress disorder** is a risk factor for the development of eating disorders that involve purging, such as bulimia nervosa and anorexia nervosa, binge/purge type. (Posttraumatic stress disorder is a psychiatric disorder that can occur after experiencing or witnessing traumatic or life-threatening events; see

Glossary.) Certainly there are also clients diagnosed with other kinds of eating disorders who have histories of sexual abuse, but as far as we know this is less often the case. People who have eating disorders and were sexually abused as children also have a much higher chance of having one or more other diagnoses along with the eating disorder. In eating disorder clients where there is sexual abuse or other kinds of victimization and posttraumatic stress disorder, these issues must be addressed to optimize full recovery.

44. Can the family environment contribute to the development of an eating disorder?

The *Annual Review of Eating Disorders* (Academy of Eating Disorders, 2006) reported that among preadolescent girls, family pressure to be thin affects body dissatisfaction more than pressure from either the media or peers. In a large sample of adolescents it was found that parental dieting or encouragement of a child's weight loss indirectly predicted unhealthy weight control behaviors.

Family influence can be direct or indirect. In a direct way family members can encourage dieting, exercise, and weight loss. I have seen a father who had a weight chart to monitor weekly weigh-ins of his 12-year-old daughter to help her lose weight, even though she was not overweight by medical charts or anyone else's standards. I have seen a father who admitted to poking his adolescent daughter with a fork and telling her, "Be careful you don't want to get too fat," because he wanted her to win a beauty pageant. Indirectly, parents may also model dieting and weight preoccupation and even eating disorders. I have seen mothers who bring their daughters in for eating disorder treatment even though they themselves have coffee lattes for lunch and green salads for dinner. I have also seen several clients over the years who had parents with undiagnosed eating or exercise disorders. I wrote my book *Your Dieting Daughter* (1996) to help parents, and others, provide an environment that counteracts the current cultural focus on appearance and thinness and fosters healthy self-esteem and body esteem in young girls.

Aside from a focus on appearance, fitness, and dieting, other factors in a family can contribute to the development of an eating disorder. As stated in the previous question, we know that childhood sexual abuse is a risk factor. There is also some research on attachment disorders and eating disorders showing that many with eating disorders have histories of attachment problems early in life. Having a good strong sense of self and a healthy self-esteem based on things other than appearance are protective factors. Parents can help instill these qualities in their children. Parents who put too much emphasis on achievements and an overfocus on external validation can affect their children's value system. Children who grow up learning to seek validation externally or value themselves only for performance and accomplishments rather than who they are may be more inclined to seek validation, praise, and esteem through appearance-related things such as dieting and weight loss.

One last note of interest in this area is the fact that research has shown that family therapy is the most effective form of treatment for adolescents with anorexia nervosa, and this may be true for bulimia nervosa as well. This tells us that families have a very great impact and can be taught to use their influence in ways that help their children overcome eating disorders. It only stands to reason then that families could also help prevent these illnesses.

PART FOUR

Getting Help

If I think I have an eating disorder,
what should I do?

What kinds of treatment are available
for eating disorders?

How do I choose a good therapist?

More...

45. If I think I have an eating disorder, what should I do?

If you think you have an eating disorder you should seek help from professionals who are trained to assess and treat these disorders. You need to get a thorough psychological, nutritional, and medical assessment. It does not really matter which professional you see first, but a medical doctor and eating disorder therapist are good places to start. If you believe these individuals are competent, you can ask them for referrals to a nutritionist and psychiatrist. See the Resources listed in this book for ideas on locating eating disorder professionals. Try not to be afraid but to think of it as hiring some professionals to help you. They will be working for you. You can interview a few people to see whom you believe fit best with you, but don't dismiss everyone while looking for the "perfect" person. Furthermore, don't wait to get started; getting help sooner rather than later may give you a better chance of full recovery. Reading through this book will give you useful ideas on understanding your illness. The information here should also help you with what treatment options exist and what you should expect from various professionals. Although it may be your inclination, I usually do not recommend that you start by reading books about other people who had eating disorders. I find these books often give people negative ideas, and many of them are actually depressing. Most clients I surveyed said that these books made them go further into their eating disorder. There are exceptions to this. *Appetites* (2004), by Caroline Knapp is one of them. Once you are in treatment you can ask your therapist to recommend books he or she believes would be good for you. On the other hand, it does help to read books like *The Eating Disorder Sourcebook* (Costin, 2007) or other reference books that can help you be a better consumer and help you understand your illness.

46. What kinds of treatment are available for eating disorders?

Treatment for eating disorders is available through a variety of professionals, levels of care, treatment modalities, and treatment programs. Usually, people start out by seeing a therapist once or twice a week. Most eating disorder treatment takes place in this type of **outpatient therapy** setting, where the client lives at home and attends sessions with treating professionals. How long a person has been ill, how severe the eating disorder is, and what medical or other complications exist determine the level of care, how many professionals are involved, and whether going to a treatment program is an appropriate choice. Levels of care and treatment programs are covered in Part Five. Treatment professionals and programs also use varying philosophical approaches to treating eating disorders. These approaches are discussed further in Part Six. The following delineates the treatment professionals who are usually included as part of a treatment team for eating disorders and a brief summary of what they provide. Information is further elaborated on elsewhere in this book.

Therapists provide psychological counseling and deal with underlying issues, body image, relationships, and specific eating disorder behaviors. Therapists should be licensed professionals or experienced licensed interns and specially trained to treat eating disorder clients. They usually work in an outpatient setting and see clients anywhere from one to four times per week. Sessions usually last from 45 minutes to 1 hour, but often therapists have longer sessions. Therapists conduct therapy in various modalities; the most common are individual, group, and family therapy. All these modalities may be included in an overall treatment plan for an

Getting Help

Outpatient therapy

Provides therapeutic intervention to individuals in need of mental health resources but who do not require hospitalization or residential care.

individual with an eating disorder. These modalities are discussed further in subsequent questions.

Physicians provide medical assessment, monitoring, and care. Ideally, you should find a physician who has experience with eating disorders. You should tell your doctor about all your behaviors and symptoms so he or she can advise you properly. Your doctor should do a thorough medical examination (refer to Part Two). The doctor should also monitor your progress and help you and your treatment team set goals. This person is in charge of your physical health, so choose your physician carefully and be honest.

Psychiatrists are physicians who are trained specifically to perform psychiatric assessments, provide psychotherapy, and prescribe medication for psychological issues. An increasing number of psychiatrists are trained in eating disorders. When looking for a psychiatrist you may already have a therapist and only need a psychiatrist to provide an assessment and any possible medication that might be useful. On the other hand, you might find a psychiatrist who can also be your therapist as well as provide assessment and treatment with medication. Psychiatrists vary in the treatment they provide and each situation is different. You need to determine what is right for you.

Nutritionists or registered dietitians work directly with meal planning, caloric requirements, weight, and other issues related to nutrition. Having a nutritionist as part of an overall treatment team has become increasingly sought after, particularly as more nutritionists are specifically trained in the treatment of eating disorders. Nutritionists should be licensed or certified (in some states this would mean being a registered dietitian) and ideally have experience treating eating disorders.

Nutritionists are trained to deal very specifically with calorie needs, providing meal plan guidance and educating you about your body and its nutritional needs and about the consequences of various eating disorder behaviors. Some are even further trained in counseling skills.

All the above professionals should work together and communicate with each other as part of an outpatient team to help you deal with every aspect of your eating disorder and help you to fully recover. Structured programs and treatment facilities provide other more intensive levels of care, described in Part Five.

47. How do I choose a good therapist?

To find a good therapist, you should look for someone with training and expertise in eating disorders. If possible, find someone who has a few years of experience treating these illnesses. Read about the philosophical approaches in Part Six to help you ask questions, determine whether the therapist is knowledgeable, and decide what you believe fits best for you. Ask the therapist his or her approach to treatment. Have an initial interview with the person to see whether he or she is a good fit and explore options to see whether someone else fits better for you. But don't let any uncomfortable feelings stop you as it will probably be difficult in the beginning to talk about your problems and symptoms to a stranger. You can also ask for references and credentials, but probably how you feel in the interview is a better guide. There are organizations listed in the Resources section that can help you find a therapist, such as www.edreferral.com.

You may also need your insurance plan to cover your therapy expenses. Hopefully you have coverage for this, and if so you may need to ask your insurance company for a list of professionals they are contracted with who specialize in eating disorders. Make sure you find a therapist on the list who really does have training and experience in this area. In some cases all an individual therapist needs to do is put his or her name on a list of providers even though he or she does not have training or experience with these disorders. If you can't find an appropriate provider, ask your insurance company for more names or permission to go to a therapist not contracted with them in order to get the care you need. A specialist in this area is extremely important. Advocate for yourself.

48. What can I expect in therapy? What kinds of topics are explored?

Individual therapy for an eating disorder varies according to the particular therapist. Therapy should include you and your therapist working on how you relate to yourself and others. An individual therapist can help you explore any underlying issues that may have helped cause or perpetuate your eating disorder. How you cope with problems and deal with emotions is all part of good therapy. The therapist should also talk to you directly about your thoughts and behaviors regarding food, eating, body image, and weight and should work directly and specifically with you on changing these patterns. If you have a nutritionist, the therapist and nutritionist should work together on these issues. The nutritionist may take the lead role with specific food-related challenges, meal plans, weighing, and so on. However, the therapist should not relegate all talk of food, weight, and body image to the nutritionist, because these are important issues in eating disorder therapy.

In treating eating disorder clients I use a very informal approach, going by my first name and sharing information when appropriate about my own recovery. I have found that most eating disorder clients appreciate this informality and in fact need to have a highly relational approach. I work from an eclectic perspective and use a variety of approaches discussed in Part Six. I use what works best with each client. I work on underlying issues and specific current thoughts and behaviors intermittently. I also use **mindfulness** exercises, visualization, and awareness training. Other modalities, such as **psychodrama** or **art therapy**, are chosen for the particular client. I believe the nature of an eating disorder makes tending to specific behavioral change important, and the attention I give in treatment to this aspect varies in degree depending on how healthy the client is. Early on in my career I realized that if treatment were left to typical psychoanalysis, clients could take years explaining their childhoods, how they get along with their parents, their inability to control their anger, or any number of past experiences, all the while continuing to exist on frozen yogurt and salad, or binging all day, or purging their dinner every night. Eating disorder clients can starve to death or have heart failure while trying to figure out "why" they are doing this to themselves. Therefore my individual sessions with clients vary greatly in nature because, along with an ongoing exploration of developmental deficits and underlying issues, I deal directly with thinking patterns, behaviors, and symptom management. Individual therapy for eating disorder clients should be dynamic and the therapist more directive than in other forms of therapy. I have trained many therapists over the years, and my experience has shown that the successful eating disorder therapist needs to take an active stance and in some way is also a teacher and coach.

Getting Help

Mindfulness

The practice whereby a person is intentionally aware of his or her thoughts and actions in the present moment, nonjudgmentally.

Psychodrama

In psychodrama, participants explore internal conflicts through acting out their emotions and interpersonal interactions in a role play situation.

Art therapy

A form of expressive therapy that uses art-making and creativity to increase emotional well-being.

In therapy I help clients gain access to what I call their eating disorder self, the part of them responsible for their symptoms, the part that is acting against what a healthy self would do. I also work at strengthening each client's healthy or core self. It is their healthy self that takes care of the eating disorder behavior. The goal is to integrate the eating disorder self back into the core self so there is no longer a separate eating disorder self acting out symptoms but rather one healthy self back in control.

The following are examples of assignments I give clients in therapy:

ASSIGNMENT:

Write all the good reasons why you have your eating disorder.

This is one of the first assignments I give, and clients are often stunned by it. They expect me to ask them to write all the reasons their eating disorder is bad or is ruining their lives or all the reasons they want to get rid of it. I explain that by writing all the good reasons, by learning why they want it and want to keep it, is a way to begin to figure out what purpose it serves. Showing the assignment to significant others also helps other people understand why their loved one has an eating disorder and why it might be so hard to give it up.

ASSIGNMENT:

Write in your journal before engaging in any eating disorder behavior.

A good way to get access to the eating disorder self and begin to deal with the eating disorder behaviors is to write in your journal before you engage in them.

Then you can bring the journal into your therapy session and discuss your thoughts and feelings you had at the time. The therapist can then help you begin to find ways to resist the behavior in the moment.

ASSIGNMENT:

Write a letter to your eating disorder.

I ask clients to write letters to their eating disorder self. Sometimes I ask them to write a thank you letter to see what the eating disorder has done for them. Sometimes I ask them to write a good-bye letter. The client may not want to write this letter because they are not ready to give it up, but this can still be a useful exercise.

I explain to the client that a good-bye letter can give us information on how he or she is really feeling toward the eating disorder. Then after the client writes this letter I ask him or her to let the eating disorder self write back so we can see what it has to say back. If they say, "I want to get rid of you, I don't want you in my life," how will the eating disorder self respond? This helps us figure out why the eating disorder self feels it is necessary to stay around.

ASSIGNMENT:

Write about your last eating disorder thought.

Clients are often thinking about their eating disorder or engaging in eating disorder behavior and yet do not say anything. Even in the middle of a session I might ask this question. I also have clients take journals home and write about thoughts they have, and then we work with those thoughts in session.

ASSIGNMENT:

Draw a picture of your eating disorder self.

I often ask clients to draw a picture of their eating disorder self and discuss this. I am continually surprised and amazed at the images clients create. I also have them draw a picture of their family at the dinner table and discuss how the eating disorder self comes out there. Artwork can be a good way to express things that are hard to express verbally.

ASSIGNMENT:

Bring food into the room.

I sometimes have a food item such as a chocolate chip cookie sitting on a table in my office. I start the session with a client with the food sitting there. Some people walk right in and say "What's that doing there?" Some people sit far away from it and say nothing. After a while into the session I'll say, "Okay tell me all the thoughts you've had about that cookie sitting there that you haven't shared with me yet." This is a way to begin to access all the thoughts and feelings a client might have just upon being in the same room with a cookie.

All these assignments help clients see that the eating disorder is not all of them but a part of them that is acting on an unconscious level they can get conscious control of.

Comments from clients about their experience of the eating disorder self and healthy self-concept follow:

> "Acknowledging a dividing line
> between the eating disorder self and
> the healthy self made recovery a bit
> less daunting. Instead of getting

bogged down by convoluted ration-
alizations and doubts, I could just
stop, simplify, use my logic, and ask
myself, 'Is this choice in my best
interest? Does it promote physical
and mental health?' Isolating the
eating disordered self that way made
it easier to defy it."

"Recognizing the eating disorder
self and healthy self is one of the key
factors to getting better, especially
for my eating disorder. It was
important to be able to recognize the
two opposite characteristics: the
restrictive anorexic self and the
bulimic self that I had within me.
Part of the recovery process involves
making the healthy self stronger so
that it will begin to take action while
the eating disorder self may just be
present but not acted on."

"The concept of healthy self/eating
disorder self has definitely been
helpful for me, especially as I have
gained more recovery and my
healthy self has become stronger.
When I notice myself thinking I
need to work out more or that I look
big in the mirror, I try to remind
myself that it is the old voice of the
eating disorder. My healthy self
knows that I am only having those
thoughts because I am stressed out
from work or I just broke up with

my boyfriend. Keeping this duality
in mind gives me a more realistic
perspective."

49. What is group therapy and is it a good choice for me?

Group therapy is very useful for the treatment of eating
disorders. A good therapy group can provide a supportive
environment where you can begin to talk freely, tell the
truth, and feel less shame about your eating disorder.
Group is also a place where you can be challenged to look
at your thoughts and actions by your peers. I believe that
most clients benefit from group therapy unless they are
very hostile or so sick or distracted they cannot tolerate
listening to or sharing with others. Groups can be very
different depending on the expertise of the therapist
running the group and the various group members, so if
one group does not work for you, try another.

By sharing with and listening to others, many people
with eating disorders learn they are not alone in their
suffering, their feelings, and their experiences. Even
though individual stories vary and people with eating
disorders are all unique, there are similarities that exist
among people who are suffering from eating disorders.
It can enhance a person's self-esteem just to realize that
he or she is neither crazy nor alone. Some clients handle
certain issues better than others, and they help each other
in this way. Furthermore, a common trait in individuals
with eating disorders is the desire to be special and
unique, and the eating disorder helps provide that. In a
group of peers also with eating disorders, clients must
explore and find other more constructive ways to be
unique. One caution is that clients in group can be

exposed to techniques for weight loss or ways to purge from other clients; therefore young clients who are seen in the beginning of their illness might be better off with only individual and family therapy.

The following is an example of what clients have to say about being in group therapy:

> "Group therapy is a place where I was able to collect other people's input and get different perspectives from what I would get in an individual therapy session. I believe group therapy provided me a place where I could talk about my issues and connect with others on a deeper level. This was an important part of recovery for me."

> "For a long time my eating disorder was very strong and I had a hard time admitting certain things. I was really lacking skills in communicating any negative feelings successfully. I was very afraid and untrusting and could even hide the truth from myself. Being in group therapy gave me the chance to take in information and to share things in an appropriate way. Recovering from my eating disorder has taken me a very long time and has required a lot of help. I know that group therapy was a very important and integral part of my treatment."

Ground Rules for Group

The therapist running the group establishes the code of behaviors or norms that guide the interaction in the group. The therapist guides the interaction by modeling, encouraging, and teaching when appropriate. The therapist helps the members of the group interact with each other. For example, in the early phase of a group I was talking to an extremely emaciated girl with anorexia who was shivering. She was quite cold, yet everyone else in the group was comfortable. I told the girl that her shivering was due to the fact that she was too thin and had no insulation or protection from the cold. Another female member of the group asked me, "Does it bother her when you say that?" I redirected the group member to ask this question directly to the girl with anorexia. She then was able to ask directly, "I wonder if it bothers you when Carolyn talks to you like that in front of us." This is one example of the therapist's function in setting desirable standards, such as a high level of involvement between group members, nonjudgmental acceptance, and a high level of self-disclosure, a desire for self-understanding, and a desire for change.

Usually, the group therapist establishes guidelines and rules for things like refraining from drugs and alcohol before group, ways that payments and missed sessions are to be handled, punctuality, and confidentiality. Therapists often bring up topics to discuss in group or lead the group in open-ended questions. At other times the therapist asks the participants to bring up issues.

The following are some topics or themes often discussed in eating disorder groups:

1. Control and helplessness.
2. Family and personal history regarding food and weight.
3. Ability to nurture and be nurtured.
4. Perfectionism, competition, and loneliness.
5. Anger and assertiveness.
6. Body image.
7. Intimacy and sexuality.
8. Spirituality.
9. Separation and individuation.
10. Acceptance and forgiveness.
11. Women's conflict around appetites.
12. Trust and mistrust.
13. Relapse prevention.

The following are excerpts taken from journal entries of clients in a group:

> "It was very hard sitting in group tonight. I just felt fat, fat, fat. And when Carolyn asked me how I felt all I could say was fat. Other people have told me that fat is not a feeling but that is what I felt. It's especially hard with the new girl. She is thinner than all of us, especially me. I bet others felt this too. I should ask them next week. This just reminds me that I will have to deal with other people and their thinness because there will always be someone thinner than me and anyway why should this matter so much. I need to find out."

"I really felt for Karen today because two weeks ago, she was so excited about her 'diet.' I knew it wouldn't last for her and sure enough, there we were today, listening to her tell us how she blew it. The diet didn't last. Now she's binging and throwing up again. I look at her and wonder what goes on in her mind. There's more to it than just being thin. She is so unsure of what she wants and who she should be. Some of the things she says just don't make sense to me, yet I have said them. Seeing her really makes me think about myself."

"I had a hard time today looking at Christy. She is so thin, it really made me feel a little sick to see how thin her legs are. She is a walking skeleton. I know we weigh about the same; this makes me have to consider how I see myself. I wonder how they all see me?"

"Just knowing that everyone else in the group is rooting for me, not judging me but supporting me to get better, has made it so much easier."

"I'm surprised at how defensive I get when someone asks a question or wants clarification about something I've said. Tonight the group members told me how hard it is for them to talk to me, especially to ask me anything because I act annoyed and defensive. I guess I always feel suspicious of people's motives and am always thinking I'm being attacked. That's how I felt in my family, exactly like that."

50. My friend is in a support group, and I am in a therapy group. What is the difference?

A support group usually means a group that individuals can attend on a drop-in basis. This kind of group meets regularly and attendees are whoever happens to come. These groups are usually run on a no-fee or donation-only basis. They are most likely not facilitated by a licensed professional (although they can be) and are designed to offer support but not therapy. Examples of support groups for eating disorders would be 12-Step groups such as Overeaters Anonymous and Eating Disorders Anonymous, or support groups sponsored by the National Association of Anorexia Nervosa and Associated Disorders (ANAD). Readers can find more information in Resources. Therapy groups are run by a professional, usually require a fee, and most often are designed so that certain individuals sign up for a period of time; thus the same group members come to every meeting.

51. What is family therapy and should my family be doing it?

I believe family therapy is important no matter what the age of the client with the eating disorder. I try to work with family members of all my clients unless there is some specific compelling reason not to. Clients often resist family therapy and give many reasons why not to do it, such as, "My family has nothing to do with this," "It will not help to work with my family," "I don't live with my family," "My family is too far away," "My parents are too busy," "My husband is too busy," or "My family has too many other problems." These reasons are not good enough to avoid family therapy. I believe some of my greatest successes in treating eating disorders have come about because of my insistence on family therapy. I have also treated many individuals who, for one reason or another, did not have family therapy and successfully recovered. Each person's therapist will help decide how and when to use family therapy. It is, however, imperative to work with family members of adolescents. For adolescents with anorexia, research indicates that family therapy works better than individual therapy alone and has by far demonstrated the best treatment outcomes. This may also be true for adolescents with bulimia, but the research results are not in as of this writing. Parents are referred to the book by James Lock and Daniel Le Grange (2005), *Help Your Teen Beat an Eating Disorder*, for a discussion of family treatment with adolescents.

Family therapy can help the clients and family members better understand the illness..

Family therapy can help the clients and family members better understand the illness. It can help teach family members how better to react to the person with the disorder and how to take better care of themselves. Family members and the client can see both positive and negative communication patterns and develop new ways of handling situations.

One form of family therapy takes place with the client and some or all members of his or her family (or significant others). Another form of family therapy is known as "multifamily group" where several families come together for treatment. I consistently hear from families and clients how important they believe both types of family therapy are in the treatment process.

The following is what clients and family members have said about their experiences:

Psychodynamics

In psychology, the study of the inter-relationship of various parts of the mind, personality, or psyche as they relate to mental, emotional, or motivational forces, especially at the subconscious level.

> "I will forever be grateful to have had the experience of sitting in a group, with other mothers; other mothers who could commiserate with me, who understood me, who had stories similar to mine and made me feel less crazy and less guilty. This helped support me to carry on again and again."

> "Thank you for providing family therapy. As a father who had no knowledge of eating disorders and who came from a culture and time that taught us not to waste anything and to clean our plate, I found the group sessions beneficial. This group allowed interaction among parents with a common lack of knowledge. It helped us discuss our worries and remove the stigma that we were the only ones who were clueless. It was a critical part of the whole process for my wife and I."

> "At first, the idea of family therapy made me uncomfortable. I didn't want to analyze our dynamics in search of some magical reason for my illness. Honestly, I didn't think

my family had much to do with my anorexia. It was, in my mind, MY illness. But, after undergoing family therapy, I realized just how limited our conversation skills were. With the safety and structure of a therapy session, we could talk and get feelings out in the open. Because so much of my struggle was about learning to express myself instead of starving, opening lines of communication with my parents and sister was essential."

"My daughter and I had stopped communicating with each other even though we lived in the same house. We thought family therapy would help us to understand our daughter's eating disorder, but it did much, much more. It helped us to understand each other and ourselves. It helped us all lead better lives.

"When our family tried to discuss subjects without a therapist, too much emotion led us into a fight. In family sessions together we learned to recognize problems for each family member: daughter and parents. A family session was a very good opportunity to listen to our daughter carefully, and recognize why and how she was suffering. During family therapy we all learned to express each feeling, emotion, and opinion we had and the therapist helped us find a common, workable, point of view. It took lots of small steps but finally we are now able to exchange our thoughts and emotions honestly."

"In family therapy we learned to communicate with each other. My wife used to be the middleman of communication between our daughter and myself, but now we all communicate with each other directly and are connected to each other for the first time. The therapist and our family formed a team to solve problems, the eating disorder was only one of them, and actually got better as we solved the others."

"Listening to the struggles between other clients and their parents and family helped me get an outside perspective about the family dynamics and most importantly for me to be able to be more empathic towards my own family. This helped me allow the staff to have my parents come to multifamily group. I was very nervous on the day of the group because, even though I had lived in the same house with him, I had not talked to my father for a year before this group. Having him come to that group was easier for me than having him show up for just a session with my individual therapist, which would have been much more intimate and scary. The other families provided a buffer, and as it turned out also a witness, for us to get past our "stand off." I think my father also felt comfort with the other fathers there in the same room with some version of the same dilemma."

"Multifamily group was helpful because it gave my family and I the opportunity to see ourselves reflected in others. For example, my dad couldn't always realize when he'd say something insensitive, but when he heard words similar to his own come out of the mouth of another father, it was enlightening. We're always a little blind to our own dynamics until we see them played out before our eyes."

"Family groups helped me in several ways. They helped me to realize that my daughter was part of a very large group of people suffering from a very real illness. I realized it was not just something in her head, that she was not just not eating to lose weight, but, for a much deeper reason. As a person who had no knowledge of this illness, I learned from the other group members how to gain information to help me help my daughter. It also gave me a sense of support knowing others were going through what we were. I gained an insight into what my daughter was experiencing by listening to other daughters speak. The personal stories helped me to understand the pain and gave me knowledge in ways I could better relate to my daughter."

52. Is treatment different for adults and adolescents?

There are differences in treating adults and adolescents. As mentioned in Question 51, adolescents should have family therapy, whereas studies show that individual therapy works better for adults. (I believe that a combination of individual and family therapy works even better and have seen this at my treatment programs, Monte Nido, RainRock, and Eating Disorder Center of California.) Adolescents have specific problems—different from adults—such as puberty or peer pressure at school or handling their first dating experiences. When working with adolescents, issues of separation and individuation from parents are important parts of the treatment. School also has to be incorporated into the process. Also, parents have more control over adolescents, ranging from what food to have in the house to being able to restrict the use of the family car. These types of control, punishment, and reward issues have to be carefully negotiated to avoid useless and damaging power struggles. Obviously, for adults there is less of an issue of someone else controlling their behaviors, although this is not always the case. I have seen couples where the husband threatened divorce if his wife would not get treatment. In treatment programs, adolescents can be involuntarily admitted by their parents, which can be quite difficult for the whole family.

53. My therapist says I need to see a psychiatrist. Does he think I am crazy?

Seeing a psychiatrist does not mean you are crazy. Psychiatrists can provide a good psychiatric assessment and help with an overall diagnosis and treatment plan. As mentioned earlier, psychiatrists are trained in psychotherapy as well as in the assessment and use of specific medicines, often referred to as **psychotropic** medications. Psychotropic medications can be helpful in treating eating disorders and other coexisting conditions, such as depression or anxiety. A psychiatrist trained in eating disorders is the best person to know what medications might be most helpful to you. Medications alone do not cure eating disorders but can be an important aspect for some people. It is important to work with a psychiatrist as one part of an overall treatment team.

54. I've heard that Prozac is useful in treating eating disorders. Is this true? Is it good for me?

Efficacy

The ability to produce a desired amount of a desired effect.

Prozac is one of a very few medications that has shown any **efficacy** in treating eating disorders, specifically bulimia. It has not proven to be effective in treating anorexia. For a time researchers thought Prozac helped prevent relapse after weight restoration in anorexia; however, new studies indicate this not to be the case. Even though Prozac has been shown to help some people with bulimia, it is not for everyone with this disorder. Studies have shown that up to 50% or more of people with bulimia are not helped by Prozac, and many more, although experiencing a reduction of symptoms, remain symptomatic on this medication. Furthermore, studies have shown that cognitive behavior therapy works just as well. It is important to consult a psychiatrist (or a medical doctor if for some reason you cannot see a psychiatrist) to find out what medication and what treatment is right for you.

55. What medications are useful in treating the various eating disorders?

As mentioned above, Prozac has shown usefulness in bulimia. Studies show that it works to help alleviate binge/purge symptoms but it rarely eliminates the binging and purging completely (perhaps only 20% to 30% of the time).

No medication has yet emerged in the research that works with anorexia. Prozac and other similar medications known as **selective serotonin reuptake inhibitors** need a sufficient amount of serotonin to work, and individuals with anorexia are lacking in this either due to starvation or perhaps to a pre-illness biological deficit in this naturally occurring brain **neurotransmitter**. Early evidence indicated that an antipsychotic, known commonly as Zyprexa, might be useful in helping clients with anorexia gain weight and maybe even in reducing obsessional thinking. However, Zyprexa is a medication with possible serious side effects, such as diabetes. Many lawsuits have been filed due to these serious side effects. More research needs to be done to determine whether this medication warrants any use. However, in seriously ill chronic cases of anorexia it has been tried, due to the mortality rate of this illness.

Topamax and **Meridia** are two new medications showing some promise in the treatment of binge eating disorder. Both have shown some efficacy in helping reduce binges, and Meridia has also shown some effect in the area of weight loss, which is not usually found in treatments of binge eating disorder. These are serious medications with

Selective serotonin reuptake inhibitors

A group of chemically unique antidepressant drugs showing efficacy in depression, bulimia nervosa, obsessive-compulsive disorder, anorexia nervosa, panic disorder, pain associated with diabetic neuropathy, and premenstrual syndrome.

Topamax

Also known as Topiramate, used originally for epileptic seizures but has shown some efficacy in binge eating disorder and bulimia.

Meridia

Also called Sibutramine. A stimulant medication and a controlled substance sold to people at medical risk due to obesity.

Getting Help

95

several side effects that should not be used unless necessary. Please refer to Part Eight, Question 96, for more information on the contraindications of using Meridia.

It is important to note that a variety of medications have been useful in specific individuals with eating disorders. However, in larger studies these medications did not prove useful across the board with specific diagnoses. Individuals vary greatly even within each diagnosis. What might be useful for one person with bulimia may not help another. Furthermore, some medications such as antidepressants might help alleviate symptoms of depression in someone with bulimia but not affect the eating disorder symptoms. For these reasons psychiatrists continue to prescribe various medications for their patients, and in many cases these medications have been useful. Your psychiatrist might prescribe a medicine for you to help alleviate symptoms that in turn will help you recover from your eating disorder.

So far, medications overall have not been very effective in curing or eradicating eating disorders. However, a few physicians believe they have found a better way. These physicians use a new form of brain wave technology to prescribe psychotropic medication specifically for each individual person rather than for diagnostic categories. This method is described in the chapter "Alternative Approaches to Treating Eating Disorders" in the 2007 version of *The Eating Disorder Sourcebook*.

56. I am a woman over 40 with an eating disorder. Is there special help for someone like me?

Older adults with eating disorders are a growing population. Margo Maine and Joe Kelly have written a wonderful book dealing specifically with eating and body image problems in midlife, called *The Body Myth* (2005); also see an article in *Primary Psychiatry* by Kathryn Zerbe entitled "Eating Disorders in Middle and Late Life" (2003). There are certain issues that professionals need to pay attention to, for example, older adults are often embarrassed about having an eating disorder because it is often thought of as an adolescent or young adult illness. They often resist treatment, not wanting to leave spouses or children at home. Older women might be more difficult to diagnose. For example, in a postmenopausal woman with anorexia, amenorrhea does not provide diagnostic help. But overall, most professionals and places with training and expertise in treating eating disorders will know how to provide excellent treatment for older clients as long as individual therapy is included as part of the program. I strongly believe that all clients should have their unique needs met by spending one-on-one time with a trained therapist. As this older population of eating disorders is increasingly seeking treatment, new programs are opening up specifically for older adults. However, I do not believe it is necessary to separate people 40 and over from other adults. In every treatment facility where I served as clinical director, I found that the older and younger adults help each other greatly. However, older adults have needs very different from adolescents or younger children and should be in separate programs from these age groups.

57. Do I need to see a nutritionist?

Sometimes a doctor or therapist is trained in dealing with the food and weight aspects of an eating disorder and can do a great job in this area. However, seeing a nutritionist allows your therapist and doctor or any other treating professionals to focus more on other issues that need to be attended to. It is also common to find that your doctor and therapist are not trained or competent in dealing with aspects of food and weight and it is helpful to find someone who can help you in this area. A nutritionist who specializes in eating disorders can be a useful addition to your treatment team. Nutritional counseling and advice can help you to identify your fears about food and weight and help educate you about the physical consequences of all your eating disorder behaviors. Most people with eating disorders have lost track of hunger and fullness, of what they like to eat, and of what "normal eating" is. A nutritionist is often the person to challenge you to eat fear foods and to help you stop food rituals. Sometimes nutritionists have meals with clients to provide support at this difficult time. Nutritionists who specialize in eating disorders know how to help you stop unhealthy eating disorder behaviors, such as food rituals, vomiting, and binging. They can also help you eat properly to avoid cravings and depravation-induced binging. A nutritionist might also prescribe nutritional supplements, such as calcium, iron, digestive enzymes, or a multivitamin. Readers can learn more about nutritional supplements in Part Ten. The nutritionist's ultimate goal is to assist you in developing lifelong natural eating patterns and making peace with food and your body.

A nutritionist will most likely be directly in charge of weighing you and dealing with your weight goals that are determined by the treatment team. See more about this in Question 60.

It can be difficult paying for a nutritionist in addition to all the various professionals recommended, especially if insurance is not covering some or all treatment. Furthermore, you may not be able to find a nutritionist, especially one trained in eating disorders, in your area. If you do live in a fairly large city and can afford it, a nutritionist or registered dietitian trained to treat eating disorders can be very useful in helping you recover.

58. What is the difference between a nutritionist and a registered dietitian?

A registered dietitian is a specific license that some states have to certify a person who has been fully trained in the area of nutrition assessment and treatment for a variety of disorders and weight control. It is important to keep in mind that not all states offer this license, and a registered dietitian license is still not a guarantee that the person is trained in treating eating disorders. When looking for professionals to work with, always try to find professionals with training and experience in eating disorders.

59. What can I expect from my nutritionist, in regards to my weight?

Your nutritionist provides a thorough assessment in the area of weight and weight control, eating and drinking habits, dieting practices, food fears or phobias, and related issues. He or she should also get family background in these areas and how your family dealt with issues of weight and dieting and other eating disorder–related areas, such as the family at the dinner table. The nutritionist, in conjunction with the rest of your treatment team, works with you to help with all the practical areas of your relationship with food, eating, and weight. He or she weighs you and helps to determine weight goals and how to reach those goals. Although not every nutritionist agrees, many believe that treatment is most successful when clients are weighed with their backs to the scale and are weaned off of weighing themselves or needing to know a number. I agree with this philosophy and have practiced this way with great success for 30 years. Scale weight is unreliable, and people with eating disorders are overly sensitive to numbers. The nutritionist and/or therapist can keep track of the numbers and communicate with you about your progress. Weighing yourself interferes with treatment. For example, individuals who have bulimia or binge eating disorder may have a good week without engaging in any binging or other eating disorder behaviors but then get on the scale and see weight gain or no weight loss, feel defeated, and then binge. People with anorexia who discover they have gained a pound get scared and usually do whatever they can to lose it. Letting a nutritionist (or whoever is serving this role in your treatment team) take over in the area of weighing and weight is a central part of recovery. The goal is to resume normal healthy eating habits and get rid of destructive ones. A number on a scale is secondary. Of course, if you have anorexia you cannot recover unless you gain weight. You will probably have to eat more food than you imagine and more than on a regular diet to accomplish this. A nutritionist can help you in this difficult endeavor.

60. I have heard about intuitive eating and the nondiet approach. What do these terms mean?

The nondiet approach was developed by many individuals who believed dieting was not a solution to weight control and caused more problems than it tried to solve. Some original writing regarding this approach includes *Breaking Free From Emotional Eating* (2003) by Geneen Roth and *When Women Stop Hating Their Bodies* (1995) by Jane Hirschmann and Carol Munter. The idea is to get away from strict meal plans and the notion of "good" and "bad" foods. The goal is to facilitate clients getting back to a natural eating pattern by helping them tune into their own hunger and fullness and their own desires, which are often completely malfunctioning in individuals with eating disorders.

The modern terminology for this approach is called "intuitive eating." In their book on this subject, *Intuitive Eating: A Revolutionary Program That Works* (2003), Evelyn Tribole and Elyse Resch claim that the ultimate ticket to freedom with food is to get back to listening to the body's wisdom. Kathryn McPhee, first runner up in "American Idol 2006," who attended my day treatment program, the Eating Disorder Center of California, reported in *People* magazine that intuitive eating helped her normalize her relationship with food, return to her normal weight, and conquer her bulimia. The following is a simple description of intuitive eating provided to me by Evelyn Tribole:

> "It's unlikely that anyone with an eating disorder can dive straight into intuitive eating. If you start too soon, without professional help, you may end up feeling scared, frustrated, and overwhelmed. Here are some of the indicators of when you are ready to move into work on intuitive eating (remember, this should be done in conjunction with your healthcare team):
>
> • *Biological Restoration and Balance.* If you have anorexia, this means weight restoration. It's not realistic to expect yourself to be able to be aware of hunger signals, let alone honor hunger and fullness. If you have bulimia or a binge eating disorder, this means moving from a pattern of chaotic eating to regular meals. Regardless of

the eating disorder, it will usually take some sort of eating plan with a nutrition therapist to get you back into balance.

- *Recognition That the Eating Disorder Is Not about Weight or Food*, but rather something deeper. Once you begin to accept this...eating will move into the realm of...self care rather than a staunch attempt at defending its existence.

- *Ability to Recognize and Willingness to Deal with Your Feelings*. As you are able to identify and appropriately cope with your feelings, the need to turn to eating disorder behaviors will decrease.

- *Ability to Identify Your Wants and Needs*. As you are able to identify your wants and needs—the less you will need your eating disorder behaviors to fill that unmet void.

- *Ability to Risk*. As your body begins to heal, both physically and psychologically, you will be ready to take and tolerate risks with your eating. For someone with anorexia, a risk may simply be eating a food without knowing its exact calorie content. For someone with bulimia it might be savoring chocolate for the first time."

Table 1, also provided by Evelyn Tribole, shows the 10 core principles of intuitive eating and how these relate to anorexia and bulimia/binge eating disorder.

61. I was told that my insurance company might not cover eating disorder treatment. What should I do?

Some insurance companies cover eating disorder treatment and others do not. Some companies cover

Table 1: The 10 Core Principles Of Intuitive Eating

Core Principle	Anorexia Nervosa	Bulimia Nervosa/Binge Eating Disorder
1. Reject The Diet Mentality	Restricting is a core issue and can be deadly.	Restricting does not work and triggers primal hunger, which can lead to binge eating.
2. Honor Your Hunger	Weight restoration is essential. The mind cannot function and think properly. You are likely caught in an obsessional cycle of thinking and worrying about food and have difficulty making a decision. Your body and brain need calories to function. Your nutrition therapist will work with you to create a way of eating that feels safe to you.	Eat regularly—this means three meals and two to three snacks. Eating regularly will help you get in touch with gentle hunger, rather than the extremes that often occur with chaotic eating. Ultimately, you will trust your own hunger signals even if they deviate slightly from this plan.
3. Make Peace with Food	Take risks and add new foods, when ready. Do this gradually; take baby steps.	Take risks and try "fear" foods, when ready and not vulnerable. (Vulnerable includes overhungry, overstressed, or experiencing some other feeling state.)
4. Challenge the Food Police	Challenge the thoughts and beliefs about food. Take the morality and judgment out of eating.	Challenge the thoughts and beliefs about food. Take the morality and judgment out of eating.
5. Feel Your Fullness	You can't rely on your fullness signals during the beginning phases of recovery because your body likely feels prematurely full, due to slower digestion.	Transition away from experiencing the extreme fullness that is experienced with binge eating. Once regular eating is established, gentle fullness will begin to resonate. Note, if you are withdrawing from purging, especially from laxatives, you may temporarily feel bloated, which will distort the feeling of fullness.

From Tribole, E. and Resch, E. *Intuitive Eating: A Revolutionary Program That Works,* 2nd ed. New York: St. Martin's Press, (2003).

Getting Help

Table 1: The 10 Core Principles Of Intuitive Eating *(continued)*

Core Principle	Anorexia Nervosa	Bulimia Nervosa/Binge Eating Disorder
6. Discover the Satisfaction Factor	Frequently, there are fears or resistance to experiencing the pleasure from eating (as well as other pleasures of life).	If satisfying foods and eating experiences are included regularly, there will be less impetus to binge.
7. Cope with Emotions without Using Food	Often, emotions have been shut down. Food restriction, food rituals, and obsessional thinking are the coping tools of life. With renourishment, you will be more prepared to deal with feelings that emerge.	Binge eating, purging, and excessive exercise are used as coping mechanisms. Begin to take a time out from these behaviors to start experiencing and dealing with feelings.
8. Respect Your Body	Heal the body image distortion.	Respect the here and now body.
9. Exercise	You will likely need to stop or at least cut back exercising.	Overexercising can be a purging behavior. Moderate exercise can help manage stress and anxiety.
10. Honor Your Health	Learn to remove the rigidity of nutrition—where there is a strict adherence to "nutritional principles," regardless of their source. Recognize that the body needs: -Essential fat, -Carbohydrates, -Energy, -Variety of foods.	Learn to remove the rigidity of nutrition. There is a strict belief as to what constitutes healthy eating, and if this belief is violated, self-loathing, purging, or other compensatory behaviors can ensue. Recognize that the body needs: -Essential fat, -Carbohydrates, -Energy, -Variety of foods.

From Tribole, E. and Resch, E. *Intuitive Eating: A Revolutionary Program That Works,* 2nd ed. New York: St. Martin's Press, (2003).

treatment but only if the eating disorder is so severe as to require medical stabilization in a hospital setting. It is important to check out insurance coverage for eating disorders when you are looking to enroll in an insurance plan. If you already have a plan and need help, you can call your insurance company for assistance with what they cover and with which therapists or treatment programs they are contracted. Also, call therapists and treatment programs directly and see if they can help you obtain coverage. Occasionally, insurance companies make single-case agreements with treatment providers not contracted with their company. This may be necessary if you cannot find appropriate help. Be sure to raise a fuss if you are not provided with adequate professionals or cannot get sufficient help from your insurance company.

You might also have a benefit for treatment but get denied because you are not sick enough to warrant the level of care requested. You may be in treatment and find out that your insurance company is saying you have to leave even though your treatment team says you need continued care. Do not be put off with initial denials of coverage. Ask to speak to supervisors, get a doctor and/or therapist to call on your behalf, write letters, and appeal any denials. It is a good idea to refuse to take "no" for an answer. Sometimes there are very clear policies and you will not win, but it is a good idea to continue to ask for a manager or supervisor to talk to at the insurance company. Continue to provide evidence on why they should cover the treatment and, if necessary, get an attorney to help you. Many cases have been won this way. You may want to go to the National Eating Disorders Association website at www.nationaleating disorders.org. There one can find information to help clients and their families fight denials of treatment coverage.

Getting Help

A federal law was passed, the Mental Health Parity Law, which mandates insurance companies to cover major mental illnesses on par with physical illnesses. Each state can decide what diagnoses are included as coverable mental illnesses. Along with illnesses like major depression and schizophrenia, anorexia nervosa and bulimia nervosa are included as coverable mental illnesses in 12 states at the time of this writing: California, Connecticut, Delaware, Maine, Maryland, Minnesota, Rhode Island, New York, North Dakota, Vermont, Washington, and West Virginia.

Hopefully the information in this part of the book has helped you with getting help. You might find that outpatient therapy is not enough to help you overcome your eating disorder. In some cases individuals try outpatient treatment for a period of time and discover they need more structure. You may already know that you need more care than outpatient treatment can provide. In Part 5 you will find descriptions of a variety of treatment settings, all of which offer a greater degree of care than outpatient therapy.

62. I have heard that I can get help on the Internet. How does this work?

The Internet is now the primary source of information for the average consumer. The National Eating Disorders Association website alone received approximately 5 million hits in October 2005. People are not only looking for information but also for services. For example, in increasing numbers people are looking for online treatment for their eating disorders.

Some physicians and therapists claim to successfully treat eating disorders on the Internet. The advantages are that sufferers do not have to drive to sessions, the cost is far less, and therapy can be anonymous. People who would not otherwise seek treatment due to shame or not wanting to be exposed might be willing to seek treatment online.

The following are the various types of Internet activity (taken from a presentation given by Kathleen Burns Kingsbury at the National Eating Disorders Association conference in Bethesda, Maryland, September 15, 2006):

- *E-Therapy*: Psychotherapists form ongoing helping relationships that take place solely via Internet communication.
- *E-Mail*: Psychotherapists use e-mail communication to supplement in-person traditional treatment.
- *Educational websites*: Often sponsored by treatment centers and nonprofit organizations, these websites offer educational material, chat rooms, and treatment referrals. (www.national eatingdisorders.org is an example.)
- *Computer-based self-help programs*: Interactive self-help programs are available on the Internet for mental health problems. (www. myselfhelp.com is one example.)
- *Telepsychiatry*: Sophisticated video conferencing systems are used to work with patients in remote locations, as an extension of traditional clinic or hospital care.

The advantages of online support or therapy are accessibility and convenience, especially for people who live in areas where there are no trained eating disorder professionals. It is also more cost effective, and often people cannot afford therapy, let alone a dietitian and psychiatrist. Also, writing through e-mails allows a client to put together thoughts in a concrete way, similar to writing in a journal, which can be very helpful. The disadvantages are that it is clearly not appropriate for severely ill or high-risk cases. Furthermore, information can be inaccurate, for example, a client could easily lie about his or her weight or about his or her identity. I knew a young man who spent hours on eating disorder chat rooms pretending to be a young woman suffering from anorexia because he met many young women online this way and was able to spend long hours in conversation with them. There are also problems with privacy and confidentiality. It is easy to look at someone else's e-mail. I once had a client whose mother got on her computer and read all e-mails between her and her therapist. A therapist once sent me an e-mail meant for her client whose name was also Carolyn. The field is grappling with legal and ethical issues regarding Internet treatment and support. Ideally, seeking help on the Internet should be an adjunct to and not a replacement for traditional therapy. Eating disorders are serious and possibly life threatening illnesses and I encourage people suffering from eating disorders to seek face to face professional help.

PART FIVE

When to Consider a Treatment Program

How do I know whether I need to go into a
treatment program?

What kinds of treatment programs are available?

How do I choose a treatment program?

More...

It is essential that the therapist, physician, and any other treatment team members agree on what constitutes criteria for a higher level of care than outpatient therapy and work together so that the client sees a competent, complementary, and unified treatment team. To avoid panic and confusion, it is useful to establish criteria for, and goals of, any day treatment or inpatient treatment ahead of time, in case such a situation arises. The criteria and goals should be discussed with the client and significant others and, when possible, agreed on before any admission. In fact, establishing guidelines for what constitutes a higher level of care is important to do early in eating disorder treatment. Involuntary hospitalizations are hard to enforce unless the person is an adolescent and for adults should be considered only when absolutely necessary.

63. How do I know whether I need to go into a treatment program?

The following are all examples of individuals who would benefit from a treatment program:

- You are a little underweight and vomiting several times a day. You have never had any treatment, but you want to go directly to a treatment program and do not believe individual therapy will be enough.

- Your daughter has been in therapy for 6 months. The therapist says they are making progress, but your daughter continues to lose weight and eat less and less at home. You want to take her to a day treatment program in your area specializing in eating disorders.

- Your wife has had an eating disorder for several years. She has been to treatment before but has relapsed. She is emaciated, weak, and addicted to diuretics and refuses to go see her therapist. You believe she is in danger and want to insist that she go into a treatment program. You feel so strongly that you might even leave her over this.

- You are normal weight, but you cannot control your exercise and occasionally you take diet pills and laxatives. You run or train 5 to 6 hours a day even when injured. You cannot eat without doing this amount of exercise and have not been able to keep a job or go to school because it interferes with your ability to do your exercise routine. You do not binge or vomit, and you are not underweight so you do not believe you are an appropriate candidate for a treatment program. However, you need structure and supervision to stop these compulsive behaviors.

An endless number of scenarios suggest a treatment program would be a good choice. It is helpful to have a qualified physician or other treating professional recommend the level of care and which program is best suited for you. There is also a list of guidelines provided here that you can check, but understand that you can choose to go to treatment anytime; it does not have to wait or be a last resort. You might have a hard time getting insurance coverage, but this does not mean you do not really need the care.

Over the years I have found that most people, even professionals, believe a treatment program is a last resort and everything else should be tried first. This may be because, unfortunately, insurance companies often do not cover treatment programs, or if they do they require the person to "fail" outpatient treatment first and/or their criteria for covering this option is quite severe. I have known clients who increased their symptoms or lost additional weight so they would meet the requirements and get the treatment they needed. I have also heard parents and therapists use a threatening tone when making statements to clients, such as "If you don't shape up, I am going to have to hospitalize you, and you won't like that." It is true that those suffering with an eating disorder often have to be "talked into" or forced by a parent or significant other to go into a structured program, but this should not be the case. A treatment program can be an excellent option, even in the beginning of treatment, and can assist in treating the eating disorder successfully early on. There are plenty of good options for this that are described later in this section.

Treatment in a structured setting, such as a day treatment program or residential facility, may be necessary when symptoms are out of control and/or could become dangerous. If symptoms are already at a dangerous level and the medical risks are significant, then a hospital or other appropriate 24-hour care setting may be required.

The following list provides indicators often used to determine the need for a residential or other inpatient setting. A hospital is necessary when a medical or suicide risk is present.

1. Cardiac dysfunctions such as irregular heartbeat, determined by a physician.

2. Low blood pressure.

3. Pulse less than 45 beats/min or greater than 100 beats/min (with emaciation).

4. Dehydration.

5. Electrolyte abnormalities.

6. Rapid weight loss or loss of 15% to 25% of ideal body weight (lower than this usually requires hospitalization rather than residential).

7. Continued weight loss (1 to 2 pounds per week) in spite of competent psychotherapy.

8. Multiple episodes of binge/purge behaviors with little to no reduction.

9. Outpatient treatment failure: no improvement or the person is getting worse.

10. Suicidal thoughts or gestures (e.g., self-cutting).

11. No support system, abusive family situation, or support system sabotages treatment.

12. Inability to perform activities of daily living.

13. Increase in impulsive behaviors such as drugs, shoplifting, risky sexual behavior, etc.

64. What kinds of treatment programs are available?

Clients often have the image of sterile hospitals, in which they are kept behind locked doors, only interacting with nurses and doctors, when they think of treatment programs. However, there are a variety of programs specifically designed to care for eating disorder clients. Some programs meet during the day and clients can live at home; whereas others are offered in homes, in a beautiful setting, with an exercise program and various other services to care for and treat the whole person—body, mind, and soul. When looking for a treatment program, it is important to understand the difference between the intensity and structure of different levels of care. The various options include inpatient hospital facilities, residential programs, partial hospitalization or day treatment programs, intensive outpatient programs, and transitional living houses.

Inpatient Hospital Facilities

Inpatient treatment or 24-hour care in a hospital setting can take place in a medical or psychiatric facility and is usually a short-term stay to treat medical conditions or complications that have arisen as a result of the eating disorder or to stabilize a suicidal patient. A patient may stay longer if the condition is severe, the hospital has a specific program for eating disorders, or there is no other facility close by offering more appropriate treatment. There are an increasing amount of good hospital programs that do have specialized staff and protocols for eating disorder patients.

Residential Facilities

Residential programs are an excellent alternative when individuals are not actively suicidal or medically unstable yet 24-hour care is necessary or desired. Many of these programs are much smaller, are in nicer environments, and feel more personal than a hospital setting and usually cost less. Many offer things that hospital settings cannot, like very individualized care, grocery shopping, cooking, exercise, and other daily living activities. This is exactly why I opened Monte Nido after having run several hospital programs.

Residential facilities vary greatly in the level of care provided, so it is important to investigate each program thoroughly. Some, like Monte Nido, offer sophisticated, intensive, and structured treatment very similar to a hospital inpatient program but in a less sterile, more relaxed, and more natural setting. Other residential facilities are less structured and provide little or no treatment or only group therapy. Do not confuse transition or recovery houses with true residential programs. Some individuals go directly to residential treatment programs, whereas others spend time in a hospital facility and then transfer to a residential program.

Partial Hospitalization or Day Treatment

It has always been clear to me that many of my clients needed more than outpatient therapy alone but did not need 24-hour care. I also realized early on that clients who have been in a hospital or residential setting often need a transitional program to help them wean off of 24-hour care. I opened my day treatment program, the Eating Disorder Center of California, for this reason. Readers can get a good idea of what a full day treatment program entails by looking up this program at www.edcca.com. Similar to day treatment are partial hospital programs, so called because they are usually a step-down level of care provided in the same hospital setting that 24-hour care is provided. Day treatment and partial hospital programs are becoming more prevalent, in part due to the fact that they cost less than 24-hour programs. Insurance companies often require them as a first step before they will authorize 24-hour care. Patients like them because they can live at home.

Intensive Outpatient Programs

Another level of care that can either be used as an initial step up, providing more than outpatient therapy alone, or as a step down from more structured care, is intensive outpatient programs. These programs meet a few days per week, for a few hours either in the daytime or evening.

Transitional Houses

Just as I opened my day treatment program initially as a step-down level of care from Monte Nido, so did I open a transition house. Many professionals like myself have found that clients do better with their recovery if they can spend time in transitional living after completing hospital or residential treatment. These programs help clients wean off of 24-hour care while still providing some guidance and structure in a home with other recovering clients, where everyone can practice relationship and daily living skills. For some of my clients this step has been essential to full recovery. Transitional living houses (sometimes referred to as recovery houses or half-way houses) are not programs to use instead of residential care, because they do not provide enough supervision and structure.

65. How do I choose a treatment program?

To choose a good treatment program you need to consider many things. If you need insurance to pay for your treatment, you need to find out what kind of treatment your insurance covers. You can also do research and select a few programs that you like and call them to see whether they take your insurance. If you have to pay for the program yourself, then you have many more options. You need to decide whether you want a program close to where you live, or whether it is more important to choose the program you believe is best suited for you even though it may be far away. There are different settings and levels of care as described in the previous question and different treatment philosophies and approaches, some of which are described in Part Six. It is also helpful to have a checklist of what to look for and what to ask when selecting a treatment program; please see the next two questions for a brief summary. Readers can find a more detailed discussion of this topic in *The Eating Disorder Sourcebook, Third Edition* (Costin, 2007).

66. What questions should I ask and what should I look for when interviewing programs?

The following list is a good guide, but choosing a treatment program is a difficult decision to make. It is important to take your time and get advice from those you trust.

Questions to ask are as follows:

1. What is the overall treatment philosophy, including the program's position on psychological, behavioral, and addictive approaches? (All good programs should incorporate a variety of approaches, but cognitive behavioral therapy to combat such things as black and white thinking, perfectionism, and irrational food fears must be among them.)

2. How are meals handled? Is there a dietitian to meet with every week? Is there supervision after meals? Is vegetarianism allowed? What happens if the meal plan is not followed? Are meal plans individualized in any way? (There should be a dietitian who meets individually with clients and flexibility in meal plans.)

3. How many and what kind of staff members does the program have? What is their expertise and training? Does the program use recovered staff members? (I believe having exposure to recovered staff is an important component.)

4. Ask for a copy of the schedule: Is there individual therapy or just group therapy? What kind of groups? Is there treatment on the weekends also?

What do clients do for exercise and recreation? Are there certified exercise staff? How much free time is allowed?

5. Is there a physician and a psychiatrist to provide treatment and prescribe medication when appropriate? (This is a must for any responsible program.)

6. How many clients are in the program? How many clients are assigned to a therapist? (Small programs can provide more individualized care and offer hands-on experience with things like grocery shopping and cooking.)

7. Who owns the program and who runs the program? (These are key people, and knowing about them, their philosophy, and their personal involvement are important. Ask to talk to the clinical director and see whether he or she has much client contact.)

8. What step-down levels of care and aftercare are provided? If these are not provided, how is this handled? (Every program should provide or assist clients in getting step-down levels of care and aftercare.)

9. How are family members involved?

10. What is the success rate? (Treatment programs should be evaluating their outcomes and be able to discuss this with you.)

67. What can I expect when in a treatment program?

Expect that when you first enter a treatment program it will be hard because all, or most, of your control is taken away and you are with people you do not know or trust. You may also find yourself in a withdrawal from your symptoms, whether you binged, purged, took laxatives, or starved. You will need to reach out and tell peers and staff what you are feeling and what is going on. You will most likely go through a number of assessments, and then a plan will be made for your treatment. If you need medical care or monitoring, that will be the first priority. You should expect to begin meeting with a therapist to set goals and work toward those goals. You will also be seeing other members of the team, such as the dietitian and the psychiatrist, to help you cover all bases for comprehensive treatment. You will also most likely attend a number of groups and have exercise and recreation time as well. Family therapy is a good idea, but you and your treatment team together should decide who will be involved. If you are young, it is critical to have therapy with your family. This is just a general overview. Each program has its own particular ways of doing things and special services in addition to the core program. Readers can visit www.montenido.com to explore in detail what they can expect in treatment at a small residential facility.

68. What is an average stay for inpatient or residential treatment?

Length of time in treatment varies greatly, depending on how ill the client is to how long insurance will pay. Usually, programs require at least a 1-month stay, but many clients need much more time than this, particularly if they need to gain weight. Some people need many months.

69. My loved one is in a treatment program. Should I be involved?

If you are a parent of an adolescent you should definitely be involved (please read more about this in Part Seven).

Generally, it is a good idea to become involved when a loved one is in treatment. The program can help you understand the person and what he or she is going through and help educate you on what you can and cannot do. You might be asked to attend a session with your loved one or even a multifamily group meeting, where clients and their significant others have group therapy. You will also get help on how to deal with your loved one both while in treatment and when he or she comes home. Be sure to coordinate your involvement with your loved one's therapist or treatment team. There are feelings you will have, stages you might go through, and things to do and not do; these are all discussed in Part Seven.

PART SIX

Philosophical Approaches to Treating Eating Disorders

What kinds of philosophical approaches are used to treat eating disorders?

What is psychodynamic psychotherapy?

Is the 12-step approach appropriate for eating disorders?

More...

70. What kinds of philosophical approaches are used to treat eating disorders?

Professionals use a variety of approaches when treating eating disorders—far too many to list and describe in this book. However, there are four main psychotherapeutic approaches to treatment that have been researched and are generally accepted as useful with eating disorders:

1. **Psychodynamic** therapy, which focuses on dealing with a person's past experiences and underlying psychological issues.

2. Cognitive behavioral therapy (CBT), which focuses on a person's thoughts and behaviors regarding food, eating, and weight.

3. Interpersonal therapy (IPT), which focuses on difficulties in relationships.

4. Dialectical behavior therapy (DBT), which is a combination of cognitive behavior therapy, interpersonal therapy, and mindfulness training (i.e., helping a person to develop a greater inner awareness).

In addition to these approaches, there is an additional often used; the 12-step approach. The 12-step program was originally developed for alcoholics and adapted for use first with binge eaters and then with other eating disorders. Please see other information that follows for more on this subject, particularly Question 75. Even though some of the following questions provide details, for a more thorough examination of the philosophical approaches to treating eating disorders, readers can refer to *The Eating Disorder Sourcebook* (Costin, 2007), in which all these approaches are discussed at greater length.

71. What is psychodynamic psychotherapy?

The origin of psychodynamic therapy goes all the way back to Freud but has changed and developed over time with many various psychodynamic schools of thought. Psychodynamic therapy is centered around the idea that certain maladaptive thoughts and thus behaviors develop early in life that are, at least in part, unconscious. The maladaptive behaviors are defense mechanisms developed to deal with problems but are not a healthy way of coping and end up interfering with a person's life in many ways. A psychodynamically oriented therapist helps patients delve into their past to uncover what caused them to develop their thoughts, emotions, and behaviors. These therapists try to help make the unconscious become more conscious, helping patients discover the reasons for their behaviors. This kind of therapy involves a patient's ability to be introspective and reflective. The idea is that once underlying issues are resolved the patient's maladaptive behaviors are no longer necessary. Psychodynamic therapy can help eating disorder patients deal with underlying issues. However, it is now generally accepted that just dealing with underlying issues is most likely not enough to resolve eating disorder symptoms, and treatment for an eating disorder must also involve dealing directly with current issues involving food, weight, and relationships. Newer forms of psychodynamic therapy, such as self-psychology, use more of this kind of approach.

Psychodynamic therapy is centered around the idea that certain maladaptive thoughts and thus behaviors develop early in life that are, at least in part, unconscious.

72. I've been told that cognitive behavioral therapy is the best way to treat eating disorders. Is this true, and what is this approach?

Over time it appeared that dealing with underlying issues may not be enough to break serious behavioral patterns such as those found in eating disorders. Cognitive therapy was founded on the belief that an individual's affect and behavior are largely determined by the way he or she structures the world, through cognitions (thoughts and beliefs) based on attitudes or assumptions developed from previous experiences. CBT is a combination of behavioral techniques and aspects of cognitive therapy. In CBT, techniques are designed to identify, reality test, and correct distorted cognitions. A common cognitive distortion of someone with an eating disorder is, "If I eat ice cream I will get fat." Specifically, CBT seeks to change this kind of dysfunctional belief and attitude to facilitate a return to normal eating and recovery. Research has shown CBT to be successful with individuals who suffer from bulimia and binge eating but so far little efficacy has been shown using this approach with anorexia nervosa. However, I have found success with clients of all eating disorder diagnoses and therefore I use CBT in all of my treatment programs; and my therapists use this approach in their individual sessions as well.

Behavioral techniques used by CBT are designed not only to change certain behaviors, but also to elicit the individual's cognitions associated with specific behaviors. CBT for eating disorders targets symptom behaviors such as binge eating, purging, and restricting behaviors. Dysfunctional thoughts about shape and weight are also dealt with directly with the goal of developing alternative thought patterns and behaviors. Monitoring food patterns, challenging faulty cognitions, and identifying triggers to eating disorder behaviors are all important aspects of this treatment.

The researched (evidenced based) form of CBT treatment is very specific and typically lasts about 20 weeks.

It is divided into three stages. Stage 1 presents the cognitive view of the maintenance of bulimia and implements behavioral techniques to replace binge eating with more stable eating patterns. Low self-esteem, extreme concerns about shape and weight, and strict dieting are all implicated in perpetuating the vicious cycle of bulimia. Stage 2 focuses on establishing healthy eating habits and the elimination of dieting. Thoughts, beliefs, and values that maintain the eating problem are thoroughly examined. The final stage of CBT is concerned with maintaining the gains made in therapy once the treatment has been terminated.

Within the first stage of manualized CBT treatment, in sessions 1 through 8, the following steps take place:

1. Orient the client, explain CBT, and establish a collaborative therapeutic relationship.

2. Get a thorough history of the individual (include eating problems, physical and familial history, prior therapy experience, etc.).

3. Introduce the idea of food monitoring sheets, weekly weighing, and homework assignments.

4. Educate the client about weight and eating, physical consequences of binging and purging, ineffectiveness of purging as a means of weight control, adverse effects of dieting, and so on.

5. Provide advice on a regular eating plan, use of alternative behaviors, and stimulus control.

6. Use significant others to bring the problem out into the open, to facilitate communication, to test the client's comprehension of therapeutic principles, and to help organize support from others.

This step-by-step list of phase 1 of CBT typifies this approach and is described in a treatment manual designed by leading researchers in the field. For more information, see *Binge Eating: Nature, Assessment, and Treatment,* Fairburn et al. (1993).

CBT is considered by many to be the "gold standard" of treatment for bulimia. This is true because in many studies of individuals with bulimia, CBT showed greater efficacy in reducing binge eating and purging behaviors than other treatments, such as medication and psycho-dynamic therapy. CBT has also been shown to be useful in treating binge eating disorder as well, and some clients even say it has been helpful in reducing weight, which is rare in treatment for binge eating disorder. However, it must be noted that in many of the studies using this treatment with bulimia, a significant portion of people remained symptomatic at the end of treatment or relapsed once treatment was over. Additionally, new research has surfaced showing that other approaches might do as well or even better, such as IPT. Therefore it seems best to use CBT in conjunction with other treatments. CBT has been studied only minimally with anorexia and so far shown some but only limited useful-ness. More studies are needed. I have found CBT effective with people who have anorexia when used in combination with other treatment modalities.

73. What is interpersonal therapy and its relationship to treating eating disorders?

IPT is a short-term focal psychotherapy designed to help clients identify and modify interpersonal problems. It was developed in the 1940s as a treatment for clinical depression but more recently is being used with substance abuse, marital problems, and eating disorders, particularly bulimia. IPT is a nondirective form of individual psychotherapy; and the specific researched

IPT protocol involves 15 to 20, 50-minute sessions over 4 to 5 months. Rather than focusing on specific food- and weight-related behaviors, this treatment primarily deals with problems and conflicts in interpersonal relationships. In IPT a detailed assessment culminating in an "interpersonal inventory" identifies core associated interpersonal problem(s) that become the focus of treatment. Three sources of information are used to identify the problems: (1) an evaluation of the interpersonal context in which the eating problem developed and, more importantly, has been maintained; (2) an assessment of the quality of the client's current interpersonal functioning; and (3) an examination of the interpersonal context of specific eating disorder episodes. Clients are helped to understand the role of interpersonal problems in the development and maintenance of their symptoms.

The treatment has three stages. In the first stage the goal is to engage the client in treatment, identify current interpersonal problems, and establish a treatment contract. The therapist and client decide which of the identified problems will be the focus of the remainder of treatment. The second and third stages are identical to IPT for depression except that with eating disorders there is more pressure from the therapist for the client to change. The eating disorder is not directly addressed, and any attempts by the client to do so are redirected by the therapist to the interpersonal context (*The Clinical Psychologist*, Fairburn, 1994).

IPT for eating disorders was "discovered" when it was being used as a control group in a study comparing it to CBT for bulimia. It turned out that even though CBT seemed to outperform initially, by the time of follow-up the clients who had received IPT were doing as well as those who had received CBT. This was not what had been expected. Other research has also shown IPT to be as effective as CBT in binge reduction in people who have binge eating disorder.

74. My therapist uses dialectical behavioral therapy. Will that help me with my eating disorder?

Dialectical behavioral therapy, commonly known as DBT, is a form of psychosocial treatment pioneered by Marsha Linehan to treat individuals with borderline personality disorder and is showing effectiveness with individuals who have eating disorders. The premise behind DBT is that some people react to emotional stimulation with abnormally high levels of arousal and take more time to return to normal. It is unclear exactly why these individuals react this way but in part may be due to a combination of nature and nurture, in other words, biological and environmental factors.

Labile

Emotions that shift rapidly.

People with borderline personality disorder and those with eating disorders, particularly bulimia, are known to be emotionally **labile** and typically find themselves in some kind of turmoil or crisis for which they do not have the skills to cope. DBT is a method for teaching coping skills and is a very directive form of therapy. DBT was originally developed to treat people who had problems with impulse control, self-destructive behaviors, volatile moods, and problems in relationships, all of which are commonly found in individuals with bulimia. Similar to CBT, DBT works on dealing directly with the behavioral symptoms. DBT also addresses interpersonal relationships and focuses on helping clients build skills in a variety of areas to deal with emotions and handle problems without resorting to self-destructive or self-defeating behaviors. DBT is often described as a way of combining CBT and IPT, and its usefulness with eating disorders will most likely be increasingly understood and accepted in the coming years. Mindfulness and awareness training are also an important part of DBT. These skills help clients develop ways of paying more attention to and becoming more conscious of their inner and outer world.

DBT has a hierarchical structure of treatment goals:

1. Reducing self-harming and life-threatening behaviors (most important).
2. Reducing any therapy- or treatment-interfering behaviors.
3. Reducing behaviors that diminish the client's quality of life.
4. Enhancing respect for self.
5. Acquisition of the behavioral skills taught in group sessions.
6. Any additional goals set by client.

Linehan's program of DBT consists of both individual and group therapy sessions. In individual therapy, through weekly therapy sessions and phone contact between sessions, therapist and client explore problematic behaviors or events from the past week in detail. Using what is called a behavior chain analysis, the events leading up to a behavior are delineated and alternative solutions that might have been used are discussed. Therapist and client examine what kept the client from using more adaptive solutions to the problem. The DBT therapist actively teaches and reinforces adaptive behaviors, especially as they occur within the therapeutic relationship. Clients are taught how to manage and deal with their emotions rather than trying to distract from them, avoid them, or use inappropriate behaviors, for example, binging and purging, to cope.

In group therapy, interpersonal effectiveness, distress tolerance/reality acceptance skills, emotion regulation, and mindfulness skills are taught in weekly sessions. Group therapists do not have phone contact with clients between sessions but refer clients in crisis to the individual therapist.

DBT groups have been an effective and popular addition in the last few years to all of my treatment programs, and my therapists are increasingly using this approach in individual sessions with clients.

75. Is the 12-step approach appropriate for eating disorders?

The 12-step approach, originally called Alcoholics Anonymous, commonly known as AA, is an addiction approach used to help those who cannot control their urges to drink and find their lives out of control because of their addiction to alcohol. The application of the 12-step approach to eating disorders came about when some individuals realized that this approach could be applied to people who had uncontrollable urges to binge on food and also felt that their lives were out of control because of their eating binges. At that time these "food addicts" were referred to as compulsive overeaters but are now diagnosed as people with binge eating disorder. The 12-step program was adapted for use with these individuals and was called Overeaters Anonymous (OA).

The OA approach offered a program of recovery from compulsive overeating using the Twelve Steps from the big book of Alcoholics Anonymous, adapted to fit problems with compulsive eating. Eventually specific OA books were written for use with this population. Similar to Alcoholics Anonymous, people in OA follow a 12-step approach to recovery and utilize sponsors—people who have gone before them and used this approach with success. Also like AA, OA meetings are worldwide, charge no dues or fees, and provide a fellowship of experience, strength, and hope where members respect one another's anonymity. For more information, see *The Twelve Steps and Twelve Traditions of Overeaters Anonymous*, Elisabeth L., (1993).

Over time, individuals with bulimia and anorexia also began being referred to OA for help with their eating disorders. Although many people with binge eating problems have found recovery with the OA approach, individuals with anorexia and bulimia (particularly those with anorexia) found this approach much more complicated and difficult to apply to their problems with food. **Abstinence** is a clear issue in AA, in which individuals must abstain from all alcohol one day at a time. The abstinence issue is much fuzzier when it comes to food. When OA first started, people who considered themselves compulsive eaters cut out foods such as sugar and white flour, and followed a plan for eating only three times a day. This is pretty straightforward, but difficult to obtain. When applied to bulimia or anorexia, the issue of abstinence becomes even more complicated. People with bulimia may try to abstain from "binge foods," but then again they could very likely binge on any food. People with anorexia should avoid the practice of abstinence since abstaining is part of their illness. In fact, OA meetings and the OA philosophy of abstinence can be problematic for people with anorexia and bulimia. The American Psychiatric Association guidelines for treating eating disorders do not recommend 12-step

Abstinence
Restraint from indulging a desire for something, for example, alcohol or food.

programs for anorexia nervosa and state that this approach is more likely to be helpful as an adjunctive treatment for bulimia nervosa. (Readers can refer to the American Psychiatric Association Guidelines and to Part Eight of this book for more information on the contraindications of 12-step treatment for eating disorders.) Eventually, different groups, such as Anorexia and Bulimia Anonymous (ABA), began to form in an attempt to meet the specific needs of these individuals. Additionally, a group called Eating Disorders Anonymous (EDA) was founded in February 2000 in Phoenix, Arizona. This group accepts all forms of eating disorders and promotes the philosophy that people can and do fully recover from eating disorders. Eating Disorders Anonymous uses the 12 steps of OA, with some additional changes and wording to encompass all eating disorders. As an example of how the 12 steps are used with eating disorders, see the following 12 steps of Eating Disorders Anonymous as taken from their website:

The 12 Steps of Eating Disorders Anonymous

1. **We admitted we were powerless over our eating disorder—that our lives had become unmanageable.** We finally had to admit that what we were doing wasn't working.

2. **Came to believe that a Power greater than ourselves could restore us to sanity.** We began to believe that we could get better, that there was a fundamental healing power.

3. **Made a decision to turn our will and our lives over to the care of God as we understood God.** We decided to trust

that as we let go of rigidity, we would not fall. As we took (and continue to take) careful risks, our trust grew—in God, in ourselves, and in others.

4. **Made a searching and fearless moral inventory of ourselves.** We looked at why we had gotten stuck, so we would be less likely to get stuck again. We looked at our fears and why we were afraid, our lies and why we told them, our shame and guilt and why we had them. (This step is the searchlight that reveals the blockages in our connection to God.)

5. **Admitted to God, to ourselves, and to another human being the exact nature of our wrongs.** We "told on ourselves." This established our authority as responsible people; we began to feel like we belonged to the human race. (This step is the bulldozer that clears the blockages in our connection to God.)

6. **Were entirely ready to have God remove all these defects of character.** We began to accept ourselves as we really were, and to take responsibility for our actions. We realized we couldn't "fix" ourselves. We had to be patient with effort, not results. We realized the results were up to God.

7. **Humbly asked God to remove our shortcomings.** We asked God to help us accept our imperfect efforts. We began to focus on what we were doing right. As we did so, the "right" things began to increase.

8. **Made a list of all persons we had harmed and became willing to make amends to them all.** We made a list of people whom we had injured or who—we thought had injured us, accepted our part, and forgave them for their part. Forgiveness brought us peace.

9. **Made direct amends to such people whenever possible, except when to do so would injure them or others.** After prayer and counsel with a sponsor, we went to the people we had injured (and fully forgiven) and admitted our fault and regret. Our statements were simple, sincere, and without blame. We expected nothing in return. Accountability set us free.

10. **Continued to take personal inventory and when we were wrong, promptly admitted it.** We listened (and continue to listen) to our conscience. When troubled, we get honest, make amends, and change our thinking or behavior. We continue to notice what we do right, and we talk about that, too.

11. **Sought through prayer and meditation to improve our conscious contact with God as we understood God, praying only for knowledge of God's will for us and the power to carry that out.** We listened (and continue to listen) to our heart. We earnestly seek to understand and do God's will, whatever that may be on any given day. We continue to give ourselves credit for earnest effort, however imperfect.

12. **Having had a spiritual awakening as the result of these steps, we tried to carry this message to others, and to practice these principles in all our affairs.** Having learned to trust at last, we share our experience, strength, and hope with others, and work to live at peace with ourselves, with God, and with life.

I know of no controlled studies showing the efficacy of the 12-step program in treating eating disorders. However, many treatment programs use this approach and many clients report that 12-step programs were or are effective in helping them get over their eating disorders. Because there are problems with using the 12-step approach with eating disorders, it is important to fully understand how this approach might fit or not fit each person. If this approach is used, there are ways to adapt it, which many professionals and sufferers have done. Readers can find a discussion of the use of 12-step programs with eating disorders in Part Eight.

76. How does a spiritual approach fit into the treatment of eating disorders?

The 12-step program includes a spiritual component and has recognized for a long time that this is an essential aspect of recovery. I too believe that spirituality is an important part of recovery, but this is something that has little or no research to support it. I also believe that healing takes place on a deeper level when there is a spiritual component. To discuss my position on spirituality in the treatment of eating disorders, I have taken information from an article I wrote entitled, "Soul Lessons," for the journal *Eating Disorders, The Journal of Treatment and Prevention* (2002).

"Superficial living is part of having an eating disorder. This is not to say that those who suffer from these disorders do not have meaningful lives. It is to say that they have lost track of the meaning. They have indeed lost track of what is really important. For example, surely a number on the scale is not more important than one's health, yet those with eating disorders live their lives as if this were the case. In the eating disorder world, fitting into a size 4 might be so important that vomiting several times a day to stay at this size is acceptable. And those with eating disorders are taking the current cultural trends to the extreme.

Treating eating disorders is a multidimensional task. Nutritional, medical, psychological, and even genetic factors come into play, and all need to be addressed. Even so, I strongly believe that in healing eating disorders we must focus not just on eradicating the eating disorder symptoms but on instilling purpose and meaning into our clients' lives. Once clients are reconnected to the spiritual, sacred, and soulful aspects of life, the need for the symptoms diminish.

Our society is not geared to help people appreciate and nurture their souls.

Our society is not geared to help people appreciate and nurture their souls. Instead, our culture focuses on external appearance and validation while our internal lives are often disregarded. In fact, at my own treatment program, Monte Nido, many clients do not even know how to respond when asked to talk about the soul or what they believe it is or what spirituality means. We incorporate nondenominational spirituality as a treatment component at all of my treatment programs. We work with clients coming from the perspective that spirituality is different from religion in the sense that religion is an organized set of beliefs and practices with set tenets for believers to follow and practice. Spirituality, on the other hand, is a more personal experience and involves each person's relationship with what is sacred and divine.

I am convinced that eating disorders represent a true disconnect from the soul. I have said many times that the eating disorder symptoms are the voice of the soul and that we must listen carefully and learn from them. At the same time we must instill soulfulness and a spiritual dimension back into the lives of our clients. When one becomes reconnected with sacredness and spirituality, the purpose for the eating disorder fades.

With this in mind, aside from discussions about God, spirituality, religion, and the devine, my treatment programs incorporate meditation, **mindfulness** training, yoga, and nature walks. We have a group we call "Body and Soul" that we use specifically to promote greater physical and spiritual awareness and how the two are connected. This group is meant to provide experiences to help clients form a greater connection to their bodies, to their souls, to other beings, to nature, to the universe, and to the divine, all of which I believe promotes spirituality and healing from an eating disorder. One concept we teach in "Body and Soul" is *Beginner's Mind*.

> *Beginner's Mind:* When I think of beginner's mind I am reminded of the movie K-PAX. The character played by Kevin Spacey comes to pay a visit to earth and takes the form of a human body for his experience here. Because he is not from earth he sees things on earth with a beginner's mind. In Zen Buddhism seeing things with a beginner's mind is a spiritual practice to cultivate.

Beginner's mind takes ordinary or common things and trains us to really look at them, notice them, and appreciate them. Imagine tasting an apple or orange for the first time if you were from another planet. Imagine describing it for the first time to your planetary friends. In fact, this is a great assignment to do with eating disorder clients. You will find them discovering that because apples are common we take them for granted instead of seeing them as this incredible life form that grows on a tree and provides succulent, juicy, mouth-watering, crisp sweetness for our pleasure and nourishment. Clients get in touch with how incredible an apple really is. We all only need to be reminded, perhaps guided, to stop, listen, and take this all in with gratitude. In K-PAX, while eating a banana, peel and all, Kevin Spacey states to a psychiatrist, "Your produce alone was worth the whole trip."

Just because we are familiar with something or it is not rare does not mean it is not awe inspiring or exquisite or sacred. The Zen concept of beginner's mind is an important concept to keep us in touch with gratitude for all that surrounds us. With beginner's mind we can look at things new and fresh. Because we have sunsets every night we take them for granted, yet this does not have to be the case.

Readers can go to www.montenido.com for more information on soul lessons mindfulness and incorporating spirituality into the treatment of eating disorders. There are an increasing number of professionals who are writing and lecturing about this subject and using spirituality as part of their treatment plans for clients. Readers may also want to consult books on the topic, such as a very light easy-to-read book using myths and stories, *Eating in the Light of the Moon* (2000), by Anita Johnston; or a small inspirational book, *Handbook for the Soul* (1996), by Richard Carlson and Benjamin Shields; or a larger philosophical work, *Care of the Soul* (1994), by Thomas Moore.

PART SEVEN

Guidelines for Families and Significant Others

Are there symptoms that will help me identify a loved one with an eating disorder?

If someone I love has an eating disorder, what is the best way to approach him or her?

Are there any DOs or DON'Ts for loved ones that are helpful?

More...

77. Are there symptoms that will help me identify a loved one with an eating disorder?

If you suspect that a friend, relative, student, or colleague has an eating disorder and you want to help, talk directly to the person, or tell someone else who can talk to him or her about the problem. Before you speak with the person it is wise to gather information to substantiate your concerns.

You can use the following checklist as a guide to what to look for:

_____ Unable to eat with others or eat what is in front of them.

_____ Cooks for other people but does not eat the food.

_____ Frequent trips to the bathroom immediately after meals (water running in the bathroom might be used to hide the sound of vomiting).

_____ Food continuously missing in the house.

_____ Becomes increasingly isolative and moody.

_____ Engages in food rituals such as cutting food into tiny pieces, chewing food and spitting it out, hiding food, or blotting food considered greasy into a napkin.

_____ Constantly reading articles or books about losing weight.

_____ Appears pale and frail, has bones showing, slight hair growth on body, or hair loss on head and sometimes even eyelashes.

_____ Bloodshot eyes and or swollen glands behind both ears (from vomiting).

_____ Highly rejection sensitive, needing constant reassurance, perfectionistic.

_____ Low body temperature, feeling cold all the time.

_____ Low blood pressure and heart rate.

_____ Loss of menstrual cycle.

_____ Stomach aches and constipation.

_____ Other acting-out behaviors, such as stealing, drug use, and promiscuity.

_____ Insomnia, poor sleeping habits.

_____ Displays rigid control around food: in the type, quantity, and timing of food eaten.

_____ Counts calories, restricts calories and avoids eating, feels guilty about eating.

_____ Weighs constantly, panics without a scale, and is terrified of gaining weight.

_____ Preoccupied with food (talks about it, concerned with what others eat, cooks for others).

_____ Food disappears in the house, large grocery bills are found.

_____ Marks on the back of hands (caused by using the hands and fingers to force vomiting).

_____ Often disappears into the bathroom or elsewhere after eating.

_____ Vomit is found around the toilet or elsewhere.

_____ Weight loss and/or preoccupied with losing weight.

_____ Tries to hide weight loss behind baggy clothes.

_____ Exercise seems compulsive and obligatory; cannot forgo exercise.

_____ Lying about eating habits, makes excuses for not eating or other eating habits.

_____ Irrational fear of fat in food and on the body.

_____ Eliminates food and food groups, only eating diet or otherwise "safe" foods.

_____ Constantly berates self after eating.

_____ Complains about certain body parts or of being too fat, or about the whole body.

_____ Eats large quantities when upset.

_____ Goes on and off diets (often gains more weight each time).

_____ Consumes lots of candy, gum, diet sodas, frozen yogurt, and coffee drinks, often in lieu of nutritious food.

_____ Hiding food, hoarding food, throwing food away.

_____ Drinks alcohol and skips meals to compensate.

_____ Constantly checks the fitting of belt, bracelet, ring, and "thin" clothes.

_____ Is using substances for weight control such as laxatives, diuretics, diet pills, stimulants, etc.

_____ Constantly eating and feeling unable to stop.

_____ Eating in isolation, fear of eating around and with others.

_____ Being afraid of running out of food, feeling like there is not going to be enough.

_____ Using food as comfort.

_____ Due to weight gain, often have similar symptoms to those with obesity, such as shortness
of breath, high blood pressure and/or cholesterol, joint pain.

_____ Mood swings, depression, fatigue.

78. If someone I love has an eating disorder, what is the best way to approach him or her?

If you are concerned about someone, the most
important thing is to show love and concern and not
criticism or judgment. You need to tell the person what
you see happening, how you feel, and why you are
concerned. It is best if you have some guidance in what
to say, and it is useful to come prepared with suggestions
for where and how the person can get help. It is
important to be as clear as possible regarding your
concerns. Contact the National Eating Disorders
Association (see Appendix B) for their brochure _How
To Help A Friend_ or other brochures to give directly to
your friend or loved one.

Even if you are a parent, do not get caught up in power
struggles or demand anything at this point, but do not
back down or give up either. It may take a few times or
a few different people before a person with an eating
disorder will listen and actually take the steps to get
help. If you are a parent, you might have to insist on
treatment and use your parental control to make this
happen. Ask yourself what you would do if your child
was using heroin. It is best to consult an eating disorder
specialist to help you in this difficult task.

79. When someone has an eating disorder, are there any DOs or DON'Ts for their loved ones that are helpful?

The following are some general guidelines that I often give significant others; but keep in mind that each case is different so it is best to consult an expert about your particular situation.

- **Don't** comment about weight—yours, theirs, or other people's.

- **Don't** weigh yourself or talk about dieting, calories, and "fattening" or "good" and "bad" foods.

- **Don't** get angry, blame, or demand; this won't help or work.

- **Don't** try to reward or punish to stop the eating disorder behavior.

- **Don't** become the food or purging police (negotiate these issues in therapy).

- **Don't** let the household be ruled by the eating disorder; get help in setting limits and other areas of this nature.

- **Don't** cheerlead: "You can do it. I know you will get better." (Cheerleading is a very common problem. It can make things worse because the person often feels that you don't understand how bad it is and may consciously or unconsciously escalate his or her behaviors.)

- **Don't** tolerate size bias. (For example, speak up when you hear people telling fat jokes.)

- **Do** love, accept, and take care of your own body.

- **Do** accept that an eating disorder is a serious illness and needs treatment.

- **Do** go to therapy with your loved one who has the eating disorder.
- **Do** get therapy and/or other help for yourself.
- **Do** educate yourself about the illness, through books and websites.
- **Do** listen and always seek to understand before responding.
- **Do** pay attention to signs and symptoms.
- **Do** be honest about what you see and feel but without judgment.
- **Do** be patient; there will be many stages you go through.

80. My wife has an eating disorder. Where can I find information about my situation and how best can I help?

People with eating disorders say that what helped them the most was the support they got. Those who have supportive families and/or spouses also tend to have a better prognosis. Get your wife help, get support for yourself, and be involved in her treatment. If your wife needs to go into a treatment program, see Question 69 in Part Five.

Those who have supportive families and/or spouses also tend to have a better prognosis.

Over the years I have talked to many husbands or boyfriends who feel left out when it comes to involvement with their spouse's or lover's eating disorder and left out when looking for resources specifically geared to husbands or lovers. Here is what a couple of husbands with wives who have an eating disorder have said:

> "I attend family groups and the therapist's comments are all geared to parents."

"I look in the bookstore and there are books for those suffering and for professionals and for parents but I couldn't find any books for me."

Providing information for spouses and partners has improved over the last few years. There are a few books out now that are geared to this situation. Interested readers should check out *Eating Disorders and Marriage* (1993) by D. Blake Woodside et al., and *Honey Does This Make My Butt Look Big* (2005) by Lydia Hanich, both written by professionals in the eating disorder field. *Eve's Apple* (1998) by Jonathan Rosen is a book written from the perspective of a man in love with a woman who has an eating disorder. This book is fiction and is not meant as a therapy book, but many men have appreciated reading this perspective, have related to it, and have been able to bring material from the book into therapy.

Aside from information specifically geared to husbands or lovers, there are other books that can help: *The Body Myth* (2005) by Margo Maine and Joe Kelly (deals with older women with eating disorders and can help a partner better understand), and *Life Without ED* (2003) by Jenni Schaefer and Thom Rutledge (helps significant others separate the person from the illness).

Much of the information in this book can be applied to your situation, for example, the medical information, checklist of symptoms, and how to choose a treatment program. However, what you really need is someone to understand you and your particular concerns. It helps to hear stories of others in your situation. See whether there is a support group in your area and/or join an organization like National Eating Disorders Association. This organization has other individuals in your same situation and can tell you how you might be able to get in touch with them through their parent Family Network or by attending their annual conference or other means.

81. What is the role of brothers and sisters in the treatment process?

Depending on age, siblings can be in therapy sessions in a variety of ways and in any event should be taken into account in the treatment process. Siblings can be very supportive or destructive and can be helped to be the former. They may also have feelings about what is going on and should be able to express them.

A young woman, I refer to only as S.D., recently spoke on a panel with me at a national conference on eating disorders. S.D. spoke about her experience as a sibling living with a sister struggling with an eating disorder. I share some of her words here as I believe they may help other siblings to think about, write about, and speak about their own experiences:

> "When my parents told me that my older sister had an eating disorder, I had no idea how big of an impact it would have on my life. I knew very little about eating disorders and their prevalence. Looking back, it now seems crazy to me that I thought this was something she would just get over and even though I was worried about her, this was probably not too big of a deal. I would worry about the things I was going to say or do because I did not know whether it would be something my sister was going to perceive as offensive.

Among my parents and my younger sister, I felt I was the hardest on my sister. I responded with more of a "tough love" approach because I felt when silently standing by I was sending a message that I was condoning her behavior. I have always been a mediator and it was hard for me to accept that I could not fix this problem for her. It was extremely frustrating to me that putting everything I had into helping her made no difference unless she was willing to work with me.

I found that being open and talking about how I felt sometimes made a world of a difference. My sister made it clear that she had no way of knowing how she was affecting me if I was not honest with her. This is where the "tough love" came into play. My sister knew that I would tell her, whether she was willing to hear me or not, how I felt and what my perspective was.

Personally, one of the most difficult aspects of the illness was separating my sister from her eating disorder. It was very hard for me not to place blame on someone or something for what was happening to my sister, my family, and my life. As I would process the emotions, I directed them towards my sister, not the eating disorder. My dad was constantly reminding me, "It is not your sister . . . it is her eating disorder. You don't feel that way about her, you feel that way about her eating disorder." Adopting this view is extremely helpful.

Because her thoughts were preoccupied with food and weight, my sister was very attentive to my eating patterns and whether or not I had lost weight. She also inadvertently made comments to remind herself and me that she was thinner than I was. There were times when these comments truly got to me and then there were times when I could ignore them and walk away. I would advise parents to be sensitive to this, knowing it might be happening and to look out for the other siblings.

I would ask that treatment professionals try to be sensitive to siblings and the impact the eating disorder is having on them, while helping them adapt to their role in the treatment team. I also think it is particularly important, in some cases, to advise members of a family to see individual therapists since representing an individual client and also supporting the family might be too difficult a task.

To parents I would say, we all know how easy it is to get caught up in the chaos of an eating disorder. The family member with the eating disorder requires so much of your attention and energy. My younger sister and I know our parents did their best to be there for us while working through my older sister's eating disorder, but this was not an easy thing to ask. It is important to ensure that the other children or members of the family have an outlet to release their emotions to. The spectrum of emotions and feelings will drive someone absolutely crazy if they are not processed, even if it cannot always be through you.

I think it is important to talk to your kids to make them aware of what is going on around them. I remember the times I panicked were the times I felt like I didn't know exactly what was going on. Keep your children informed and to your best ability, try to keep as little secrets as possible.

To other siblings going through this I want to say that it is so important to know you are not alone with the range of emotions you will feel and it is absolutely normal. No matter how hard you try, you will feel and think things that you wish you weren't feeling or thinking. There were times that I could not stand to look at my sister because I was so angry that she refused to get better and there were times that it hurt so badly all I wanted to do was cry for her. It used to make me feel so guilty, like I was a horrible person, for not empathizing with my sister.

It took me some time to realize this is normal and just part of processing the emotions of the experience.

Again, I want to stress the importance of separating the illness from the individual. It might take some time because this is a hard thing to do, but it is essential if you want to keep your relationship with your brother/sister.

My younger sister and I both found that it was hard as siblings to assume the responsibility of parental oversight or supervision for a sibling with an eating disorder. Sometimes you might feel that you are being asked to be responsible for things you are not capable of or that you are being held accountable when you shouldn't be. Be honest with your parents if the burden is too much; they might not know unless you share it with them.

I was adamant about not letting my sister completely off the hook. It is important to make it clear that there is accountability for getting well and you will help however you can but you cannot do it for him or her. It is also important for you to realize as a sibling there is only so much you can do without his or her cooperation.

For Everyone: I think it is extremely important to keep the focus of every day life off of food. I realize this is difficult because I remember my sister was constantly talking about food, asking when and what the next meal was, and even calculating calories. When this is the environment you are living in, it becomes hard not to become preoccupied yourself. This can develop into a dangerous pattern.

I believe the attitude of "one day at a time" was key in helping my family through the hardest of times. There is only so much you can take on at one time and there is only so much you can face in 24 hours. Take it one day at a time. It has been proven that eating disorders are curable. The more we know, the better our chances are of fighting it. Keep hope for recovery and remember there is help out there.

The information provided by S.D. gives a good overview of the issues siblings face. However, each case is different, so ask the advice of a therapist or treatment team as how best to include and help brothers and sisters.

82. Are there specific books for family members or significant others to read?

There are many books now available for family members and significant others. Some of these are listed in Question #80. There are some books that tell stories, some offer advice, others are sad commentaries on unsuccessful treatment. All books listed in Resources should be helpful. My own books, *Your Dieting Daughter* (1996) and *The Eating Disorder Sourcebook* (1999), have been highly rated by loved ones as well as clients. A few others worth mentioning here are *Surviving an Eating Disorder* (Siegel et al., 1997), *Because I Feel Fat* (Paulson and McShane, 2004), *Eating Disorders: A Parent's Guide* (Bryant-Waugh and Lask, 2004), and *Help Your Teen Beat an Eating Disorder* (Lock and Le Grange, 2005). Keep in mind that no book can adequately cover your personal situation. Furthermore, these books are each a little different so you will find conflicting advice if you read them all. Therefore, it is necessary to have trained professionals helping you with your unique situation.

83. My mother was diagnosed with an eating disorder. What can I or should I do?

If you are the child of a parent who you know or suspect has an eating disorder and you have no idea what to do, call a professional organization like the National Eating Disorders Association for help. You can also look in the phone book or on line for local eating disorder organizations or professionals to talk to and get guidance. If nothing else, find another responsible adult to share your situation with.

It is very difficult when a parent is diagnosed with any illness. Depending on your age and the severity of your mother's or father's eating disorder, there are several things you can expect. Because as the child (whatever your age) you are not the one in charge, there may be very little you can do. But as mentioned earlier, you should talk to someone. Hopefully you will be included in therapy sessions and be told what is going on. Hopefully you will have another parent who is making sure your whole family is getting appropriate help. There are very few resources geared specifically to children of those with an eating disorder, but there is a good book written by Daniel Becker, *This Mean Disease* (2005), about his experience growing up with a mom who had an eating disorder. It is a sad story because Dan's mother died, but the book may help others feel not so alone and help put words to their thoughts and feelings. Dan is also a positive man and does offer messages of hope. Of course, the book is not appropriate for very young children. Hopefully a therapist can help very young children express their thoughts, fears, and feelings.

84. My adolescent daughter has bulimia and is in treatment. Am I supposed to be involved?

You should definitely be involved in your daughter's treatment. Research shows that family therapy is the most successful form of treatment for adolescents with anorexia, and there is already indication that this may also be true for adolescents with bulimia. If a therapist or treatment team does not include you in the treatment, find another one, unless you are so sick yourself or there is some other problem indicating that your involvement would be harmful. I have never met a parent who was sorry that he or she had gotten involved too soon, but I have met many who suffered greatly for getting involved too late. You have a lot to learn about the illness and about how you can help. Listen to trained professionals who come recommended and do not try to call the shots without some help and advice. Keep in mind that this whole experience will be very hard on you, and you need to get help for yourself.

85. If I live with someone who has an eating disorder, should I throw away my scale?

Absolutely, throw out your scale, not just because of the person with the eating disorder but because you have no need for one yourself. Numbers on scales can be misleading. Scales are an unreliable measure of health and cause more harm than good. If you need to lose weight for medical reasons, get help to develop an appropriate way of eating and exercising that you can do for life and focus on health not weight. You'll eventually know if you are losing weight in the long run and in any event short term success means very little anyway. Remember there was a time before we had scales. People were able to keep fit and healthy without them. In fact, we have more obesity now than ever before with all of our scales, diet food, and diet supplements.

Remember there was a time before we had scales.

86. My loved one has an eating disorder but I know I need help for myself. What should I do?

It is wise to seek help for yourself when a loved one has an eating disorder. The stronger and healthier you are, both physically and emotionally, the better you will be at helping others. You will have many feelings in this process: You may get angry, feel neglected, not know what to do, or need someone you can talk to for guidance. There are good therapists who know how to help. It is best to find someone who understands eating disorders, because you will be looking to this person for guidance and understanding in regards to your feelings, responsibilities, and overall relationship with the person with the eating disorder. You might also find help at a support group for significant others but these are hard to find. Consider asking the person who is treating your loved one for referrals. If you do see a therapist, it is beneficial for your therapist and your loved ones' therapist to collaborate. Lastly, you might find benefit from joining The National Eating Disorders Association. This organization includes significant others in its mission to help in the fight to cure and prevent eating disorders. There are several opportunities to get information, get help, and get involved.

87. My child just got out of an eating disorder treatment program. What do I do now?

If your child was just discharged from a treatment facility, the staff there should have given you a very specific aftercare plan to follow. If they did not do this, you should call them and ask for a meeting in person or on the phone to get a plan and referrals for an aftercare treatment team and for guidance as to your continued involvement. At Monte Nido, we have our clients start sessions with their aftercare team before leaving our program. I tell parents and spouses that one of their main jobs, aside from offering support (a listening ear and love), is to make sure the person stays in treatment. Sometimes clients believe they don't need the aftercare, sometimes they start but find a myriad of excuses not to continue, and sometimes they don't like their therapist or other treatment professional and fire them without having new ones in place. I have also seen parents who were of the mindset that a treatment program would "cure" their daughter and were skeptical of the need for aftercare. As a parent of a child or adolescent, you have control and can make sure your child stays in therapy. Make sure you are also included. Ongoing family therapy is critical. If you are a parent of a young adult, you probably still have a great deal of control, both financially and emotionally. If your adult child refuses to continue treatment, you may need to stop supporting them financially, even stop paying for school. Ask yourself what you would do if he or she were a heroin addict. Even if your child is a young adult, insist on being included in the treatment. I believe family sessions are crucial, but if your child is away at school or there are other reasons you are not included in the sessions, at the very least insist on treatment update reports on your child's progress and health status. If you are the parent of a child who is much older, for example, in their thirties, you can also offer support and go to therapy sessions. Try to be included in his or her therapy even if only minimally to better understand the situation and to get guidance on how best you can help.

88. I felt good when my family member got help, but sometimes I get angry or lose hope. Is this normal?

It is normal to go through many emotions during this process. Eating disorder treatment usually takes a very long time, and feelings of frustration and despair are common. In the book, *Eating Disorders: Nutrition Therapy in the Recovery Process* (1997), Dan and Kim Reiff delineate six stages that parents, spouses, and siblings go through. I find that sharing these and talking about them with significant others is helpful. I list the stages here and provide a brief summary of the kinds of things these stages represent.

Stages of growth experienced by family members after becoming aware that a person they love has an eating disorder:

STAGE 1. DENIAL: It is unfortunate that people wait too long to get help, believing that it is just a phase or "My daughter is so smart she will figure this out." Once it has been accepted that there is a problem, there is almost always denial of how serious it is.

STAGE 2. FEAR, IGNORANCE, AND PANIC: Finding out is often a shock. It is difficult to be unprepared and uninformed, not knowing what to do or where to get help. This can lead to inappropriate initial responses, such as "Why can't you just stop?" or "I am leaving you, if you don't stop." or "You look fine to me."

STAGE 3. INCREASING REALIZATION OF THE PSYCHOLOGI-CAL BASIS FOR THE EATING DISORDER: Family members and significant others begin to understand the complex nature of eating disorders. They become involved in the treatment process and look at their own roles in the development or perpetuation of the eating disorder. They increasingly learn more appropriate ways to respond to all kinds of situations

STAGE 4. IMPATIENCE/DESPAIR: After a while loved ones often begin to feel that progress is slow. They might get angry or feel overwhelmed and frustrated, even hopeless. This is a time when family members and significant others need to be shored up, offered additional support, reminded that treatment may take years. I ask some other parent or spouse who has been through the same thing with a loved one who is now recovered to talk with parents in order to offer empathy, encouragement, and hope. This is the time for a significant other to begin to work on acceptance and shift the focus from the person with the eating disorder to oneself.

STAGE 5. HOPE: When significant others can be shown or can see on their own even small signs of progress in the person with the eating disorder, hope comes back. With proper help, significant others can find hope even if it is in how they themselves are doing. At this point it becomes possible to develop a healthier relationship with the person with the eating disorder.

STAGE 6. ACCEPTANCE/PEACE: Whether the person with the eating disorder is recovering, recovered, or never gets better, significant others will hopefully find peace and acceptance. Acceptance and peace may be hard to achieve—especially under certain circumstances—but are essential for optimal well-being. A great example of this is that of Doris and Tom Smeltzer, whose daughter Andrea died one year after being diagnosed with bulimia. After their initial grieving and what they would call an "awakening," Doris and Tom created a website, www.andreasvoice.org. Doris and Tom speak around the country helping bring awareness through the story of their own suffering and transformation. Using some of Andrea's own words from excerpts of her diaries, Doris also wrote *Andrea's Voice—Silenced by Bulimia*

(2006), a sensitive and compelling book about understanding, love, grief, and acceptance. This book delineates the pressures of being a parent or a child in a climate where the pursuit of thinness is the norm. Doris seeks to open hearts and minds as she describes emotions and transitions that loved ones of those with eating disorders go through, all the while looking at her own responsibility in Andrea's condition. As I wrote in the book's forward, "Without blame or judgment, Doris seeks to find cause and responsibility to heal not just herself from the loss of her daughter, but society in general from the loss of something much greater." Even with the most devastating outcome, Doris and Tom are examples of finding peace and acceptance not only for themselves but spreading it to others as well. They both agree that Andrea's eating disorder was a teacher but with lessons they wished they had learned sooner. To learn more about Tom and Doris and the Andrea's Voice Foundation, or to schedule a presentation with Tom and Doris, or just to get more resources and information, contact www.andreasvoice.org.

PART EIGHT

Getting Better

Can you be recovered from an eating disorder?

What does the term "recovered" mean?

My therapist uses the term "recovering" from an eating disorder. How is that different from "recovered"?

More...

89. Can you be recovered from an eating disorder?

Many people, including myself, have recovered fully from their eating disorders. In fact, most of the staff members at my treatment programs are recovered. I have treated countless people over the last 30 years who are now recovered. Research shows that although it takes several years, most people with eating disorders can be recovered. Not everyone will become fully recovered, but I hope that soon there will be no more questioning as to whether most people can be.

90. What does the term "recovered" mean?

There is no standard definition of what "recovered" means; even researchers use varying definitions. One definition used is when the person no longer meets the diagnostic criteria. The problem with this is that a person who once suffered from anorexia or bulimia but no longer meet the full criteria can still be very symptomatic. Being recovered to me is when the person can accept his or her natural body size and shape and no longer has a self-destructive or unnatural relationship with food or exercise. When you are recovered, food and weight take a proper perspective in your life, and what you weigh is not more important than who you are; in fact, actual numbers are of little or no importance at all. When recovered, you will not compromise your health or betray your soul to look a certain way, wear a certain size, or reach a certain number on a scale. When you are recovered, you do not use eating disorder behaviors to deal with, distract from, or cope with other problems.

When you are recovered, you do not use eating disorder behaviors to deal with, distract from, or cope with other problems.

91. My therapist uses the term "recovering" from an eating disorder. How is that different from "recovered"?

The term "recovering" was originally used in the 12-step program of Alcoholics Anonymous and later adapted for use with all kinds of other "addictions" and behaviors including eating disorders. Sober alcoholics and other addicts refer to themselves as "recovering" even if they have been abstinent from drugs and alcohol for years. The reason for this is that these illnesses are considered addictions and diseases from which one can never be fully recovered. In other words, the addict or alcoholic must forever abstain from these substances or they will relapse. People in Overeaters Anonymous followed suit. Even though eating disorders can seem a lot like addictions, many professionals do not see them in this light. Eating disorders are not considered addictions by the American Psychological Association (APA) Guidelines or the Academy of Eating Disorders. There is no evidence that eating disorders are caused by an addiction to food. Obviously people with eating disorders cannot have the goal of abstaining from food. Furthermore, it can be detrimental to try to abstain from particular kinds of food (unless there is a health reason to suggest otherwise). Restricting food intake can be a set up to binge. For some people the guilt and/or desire to nullify the consequences can lead to purging what was consumed. The bottom line is that people with eating disorders have to learn to deal with food every day and in fact several times a day and this is vastly different than eliminating alcohol out of your life if you are an alcoholic.

The bottom line is that people with eating disorders have to learn to deal with food every day and in fact several times a day and this is vastly different than eliminating alcohol out of your life if you are an alcoholic.

Getting Better

The 12-step approach is derived from a disease model. Alcoholism is seen as a brain disease, and alcoholics cannot drink because their brains are different. Because of the new research in genetics and brain scans, an increasing number of people believe that eating disorders are diseases. In fact, The National Institute of Mental Health recently declared anorexia nervosa a brain disease. It is important to note that changes in the brains of those with anorexia may, at least in part, be due to the illness itself. Anorexia and all of the eating disorders are serious illnesses that deserve medical and psychological intervention; and if calling them diseases helps us all (including insurance companies) to appreciate their legitimacy, then I am eternally grateful and supportive. However, there are some potentially serious ramifications to this view. Too often these days I hear eating disorders being compared with breast cancer or leukemia. These are medical diseases not considered to have psychological origins. We would not ask a person with breast cancer to go for psychotherapy to help her understand the reasons for her cancerous behaviors. We would not ask cancer sufferers to try to heal their disease through the use of cognitive behavioral therapy. Yet, therapy does work with eating disorders. Recently, a prominent physician who holds the diseased brain view postulated that therapy for eating disorders will become obsolete when medications are found to treat the brain disease. After 30 years in this field I find the quick fix, cure in a pill, solution difficult to swallow (pun intended). Even if there is symptom remission, will true healing take place? These are necessary discussions we must continue to explore in the field. Meanwhile, therapy for people with eating disorders can be successful and has helped thousands of people to get better and fully recover. As mentioned earlier in this book, family therapy for adolescents with anorexia has been shown to be successful up to 80% of the time. Family therapy will not cure leukemia. If we follow the disease model too closely, we might minimize a person's personal responsibility in recovering from their eating disorder. Furthermore, we might find ourselves once again telling individuals who have eating disorders that they cannot be recovered but only recovering or "in remission." This would be selling them short and not accurately representing the truth.

I respect anyone who found his or her recovery in a 12-step program. I have worked with great therapists who got over their eating disorder using the 12-step approach. I'm not against the 12-step program for everyone; there are valuable aspects to it, but caution must be advised when applying it to eating disorders. For a full discussion of this topic, readers can refer to *The Eating Disorder Sourcebook, Third Edition* (Costin, 2007).

92. Can you die from an eating disorder?

Most people who suffer from an eating disorder do not die from it. However, many people do die from eating disorders. Some die from the medical complications, and others take their own life after years of ceaseless suffering. What we do know tells us that anorexia nervosa is known to be the most fatal of any psychiatric illness, with a substantial risk of death and suicide. In fact, the mortality rate associated with anorexia nervosa has been reported to be 12 times higher than the death rate of all causes of death for females aged 15 to 24 years. A study reported in the *International Journal of Eating Disorders* in 2000 found that features correlated with fatal outcome are: longer duration of illness, binging and purging, **comorbid** substance abuse, and comorbid

Comorbid

Coexisting; in medicine and in psychiatry, *comorbidity* refers to (1) the presence of one or more disorders (or diseases) in addition to a primary disease or disorder and (2) the effect of such additional disorders or diseases.

affective disorders. Research on actual death rates for anorexia varies depending on the study. A study by the National Association of Anorexia Nervosa and Associated Disorders reported that 5% to 10% of those with anorexia die within 10 years after contracting the illness, 18% to 20% will be dead after 20 years, and only 30% to 40% ever fully recover. Consequently, it is often cited that as many as 20% of those with anorexia die; however, other studies have shown this figure to be inflated.

The mortality rate for bulimia is even harder to determine from existing data. Most statistics on mortality in eating disorders are about anorexia. What is published suggests that the mortality rate for bulimia is much lower than for anorexia. A 1997 study in the *American Journal of Psychiatry* reported the mortality rate for bulimia to be approximately 0.3%. Figures regarding mortality rates for Eating Disorders Not Otherwise Specified including binge eating disorder are not readily available.

One problem with assessing mortality rates is that people who die from an eating disorder rarely have the eating disorder listed as the cause of death. Instead of anorexia nervosa, a death certificate may read myocardial infarction, even though it was caused by anorexia nervosa. The same is true for bulimia. In fact, at a 2006 National Eating Disorders Association conference in Bethesda, Maryland, it was reported that perhaps more people die from bulimia nervosa than from anorexia nervosa, but the deaths are listed as heart failure. This is a problem that the eating disorder field is trying to change.

93. What is the prognosis (expected outcome) for people with eating disorders?

Treatment outcomes are different for various illnesses and age groups, but an overall summary can be provided here, taken from various sources. Readers can consult Pamela Keel's book, *Eating Disorders* (2004), and Rachel Bryant-Waugh's book, *Eating Disorders: A Parent's Guide* (2004), for more information.

Anorexia nervosa is the most tenacious and difficult illness to treat. Family therapy has shown the best treatment results for adolescents, and the use of family therapy may improve our current situation regarding overall treatment results. Overall surveys show that about two-thirds of children and adolescents make a good recovery. This means they return to a normal weight, menstruate, lose their preoccupation with weight and shape, and lead normal lives. The majority of the remaining third make a partial recovery, which usually means being able to live a fairly normal life even while keeping a weight that is too low, continuing to obsess about food and weight, and irregular or no menstruation. A small minority (around 5%) of young people with anorexia will continue to do poorly, and some of them will even die.

Although there are discrepancies in the research, most evidence suggests that the longer the person has had the illness and the older the age at onset, the more likely that the treatment will be long and chronic with poorer results. Most studies suggest that somewhere around 30% to 40% of those with anorexia fully recover, 30% to 40% will be in and out of treatment with a fair outcome, and 20% to 30% will have a poor outcome. Remember

Getting Better

that these figures do vary depending on the study. A long-term study out of UCLA showed that after two years no one had fully recovered but approximately 80% of the clients had recovered by the 10-year mark, and the new family therapy of adolescents with anorexia (with an illness duration of less than three years) shows an approximate 80% recovery rate in the first year. Our treatments are getting better.

Bulimia nervosa, when treated properly, can have a good prognosis. It is important to note that clients with bulimia are often still symptomatic after treatment, but the symptoms are reduced. Specific treatments, like CBT, designed to target binge/purge behaviors, have shown a significant reduction in symptoms in 75% to 85% of adult clients; but these levels fall over time post treatment. Other treatments like IPT and DBT have also been shown to be effective. Using medication may enhance positive results. We do not have enough data yet for adolescents. Current studies are underway to determine whether family therapy is the treatment of choice for adolescents with bulimia. Relapse is common with bulimia, and clients might need several treatment attempts. Looking at results from a number of studies, it seems that approximately 50% of individuals with bulimia recover and maintain their recovery; 30% improve but remain symptomatic; and 20% continue to meet the full criteria, but after 10 years this drops to about 10%.

As for Eating Disorders Not Otherwise Specified and binge eating disorder, there is not much known about the long-term course, and more research needs to be done before we can realistically discuss outcome rates. Two studies of individuals with binge eating disorder at five or more years following presentation with the illness showed that approximately 52% in one study and 82% in the other were improved or recovered.

94. Are there things that are indicative of a better treatment outcome?

Researchers have pointed to characteristics shown to lead to a better outcome:

- A good support system, family and/or otherwise
- A good social life.
- Early intervention when a problem arises, whether in an adult or child.
- Illness and treatment beginning at a young age.
- Family therapy, if an adolescent.
- The eating disorder does not involve purging.
- Alcohol and drugs are not involved, especially in anorexia.
- The client establishes a positive alliance with the therapist.

In addition to the previous list, I have found several other things that contribute to a good outcome. One of these things is the experience of working with someone who has recovered. Almost without exception, clients from my private practice and those from my treatment centers report that working with one or more professionals who recovered from the disorder was one of the big factors in their getting better.

The following quotes are indicative of what clients say about this factor:

"For me personally working with a therapist who was recovered from an eating disorder was the only way that I could feel safe being honest about my behavior, which felt shameful, misunderstood, and irrational, as well as something I desperately needed. I didn't believe that anyone could possibly understand or help me and this fear prevented me from getting help for more than ten years. When I learned that recovered women were working at the treatment center and that my therapist was recovered, it gave me hope for the first time that maybe I could get well after so many years of being sick. It is very hard for me to be honest about my feelings and to trust people; and having the eating disorder was making me more and more disconnected from others and myself. Knowing that my therapist could understand things about having an eating disorder and the slow process of recovery helped me feel less alone and also really understood for the first time in my life probably. I am a very functional person who wears a very convincing mask. For me personally, the recovered staff where I was in treatment were not only instrumental in my recovery process, but also the reason that I agreed to go in the first place."

"While in treatment I found that having a staff of recovered professionals gave me a sense of hope, which alone I was unable to muster. Working with a therapist who had actually been to hell and back brought a sense of perspective into my situation that "back" was indeed an option. Because I was able to identify with my therapist I was also able to envision my own path back to health. Also the concept of having a large group of people who had been involved in the same whirlwind disorder and dysfunction made my eating disorder mind feel less unique, less empowered, and less desirable. I was no longer the only tortured soul. I was in a house full of souls that were old and wise and had certainly seen their fair share of torture. I saw the staff as reborn and empowered. It made me want that too."

"Recovery in any sense is a huge decision and commitment. In the past, I had never actually seen anybody recover, so as much as I wanted to get over my disorder, or as sick as I knew I was, I couldn't comprehend how I would be able to work so hard and give up something so important to me, if there was no real way to recover anyway.

Dealing with recovered staff has given me the motivation I wasn't capable of finding inside myself. When I was feeling absolutely horrible in the beginning stages of recovery, to hear someone who I admire and respect tell me that they had gone through a similar feeling or situation and by persevering they are now on the other side of life, helped me realize this feeling was only temporary. To be able to see that people have been in pain, but they have pushed through it, and they are now some of the healthiest, wisest people I have come across in my life—that is what made the difference for me. To make the commitment in my recovery, I needed more than a leap of faith, I needed to know that there was a reason, that there is a life on the other side that is more rewarding than what the eating disorder allowed me, and that it is worth the pain of the recovery process to get there."

A few other factors I have found that contribute to successful recovery came from a survey I once conducted of former clients. I discovered that for the most part those who had recovered had 3 things in common:

- They were not weighing themselves.
- They were writing in a journal.
- They reached out for help at the first sign of a problem.

173

These are seemingly simple tasks but often hard for those with eating disorders to do. I stress the importance of these behaviors to all my clients since those who are recovered used them in their successful journey.

95. How long does treatment take?

Research has shown that full recovery from an eating disorder takes a long time and can even take 7 to 10 years. I have seen clients get better much sooner, even within a year. I have also seen clients who today, well after 10 or 15 years, still have an eating disorder. It is very difficult to determine who will get better and how long it will take. Some features have been shown to lead to a poorer or a better prognosis; refer to Question 94. It is best to assume that you, or your loved one, are in for a long haul, at least a few years. A huge mistake is often made in not staying in treatment long enough. Symptom reduction, or even abstinence, is not enough for a full recovery. Parents too often listen to their child who pleads to let her or him go back to sports or college, quit therapy, and get on with life. Husbands want their wives and the family back to normal. Eating disorder individuals are often very bright and accomplished, and parents or spouses readily believe that their child or spouse can apply this capability to recovery, thus being able to get over the illness readily. This is not necessarily the case, and parents and spouses must pay heed to the fact that eating disorders are tenacious illnesses. Loved ones should take seriously what treatment professionals recommend. It is better to err on the side of caution. Extra time in treatment will not have as **deleterious** consequences as relapse.

Deleterious

With a harmful or damaging effect on somebody or something.

96. I have been treated for binge eating disorder and have successfully abstained from binging for over six months but I have not lost weight. Is this really successful treatment?

The issue of weight loss and binge eating disorder is a very problematic one. Weight and binging are interconnected, yet a person can be considered recovered from binge eating disorder if he or she no longer binges even if the weight remains high. There is no weight criterion for the diagnosis; a person can be overweight or obese and not have an eating disorder. Most research indicates that treatments for binge eating disorder have fallen short in the area of weight loss, although there is a new medication, Meridia, which has shown some promise in this area. Be aware that Meridia is a stimulant medication and a controlled substance that is only supposed to be sold to people who are at medical risk due to their obesity. This medication has serious side effects, such as nausea, constipation, dizziness, drowsiness, menstrual pain, and even increased appetite and thoughts of suicide in some people. You can also become physically and psychologically dependent on this medication. Several other medications of this kind originally on the market for weight loss have been taken off the market, so it is wise to be cautious. If used at all, Meridia should only be used under a doctor's supervision. I have treated many people with binge eating disorder who, over time, have lost weight without medication. It is important to work with professionals who help support and encourage you on the work you have done to overcome your eating disorder. It is also important to have professionals who can help you look at the issue of weight loss and your health to determine whether it is really necessary for you to lose weight or whether you are struggling to attain a weight that is unnatural for your body. It might be good for you to connect with people from Health At Any Size (see Resources). If you find that you really do need to lose weight, I suggest you work with a professional who can help you with what is right for you. There are many professionals who use a nondiet approach such as described in the book *Intuitive Eating* (2003) to help find your healthy weight and protect you from being triggered into binge eating.

97. Are there certain phases of the recovery process?

Clients go through many phases of recovery. In the beginning clients are unaware of how bad the eating disorder is or could become. Clients often hold back telling the truth about everything they are doing or feeling. As treatment progresses, clients should begin to get a better understanding of what it will take to get better and why they have their illness. Most clients will not be able or perhaps even willing to give up their symptoms right away and usually give up behaviors bit by bit. Sometimes there are long plateaus in treatment and the recovery process. I have also never seen a person follow a straight road to recovery; usually there are slips and lapses and even relapses in their progress. It is important to keep in mind that symptom reduction or even abstinence does not mean full recovery. Clients can hold back from engaging in symptoms, but if they have not resolved the "issues" that caused or perpetuate the eating disorder, they are not likely to remain symptom free. It is important to note that what I mean by "issues" does not just refer to things that happened in the past. An issue could be the inability to deal with a highly anxious temperament or the lack of impulse control. Dealing with causal underlying issues does not mean Freudian analysis.

Getting Better

PART NINE

Preventing Eating Disorders

Can eating disorders be prevented?

Is there anything I can do to prevent eating disorders?

More...

98. Can eating disorders be prevented?

We finally have a better understanding of what eating disorders are and what causes them. To prevent eating disorders, we need to look at all contributing factors that go into the making of these illnesses. Biological researchers will continue to try to find biological or genetic causes and develop medications that may help prevent as well as treat eating disorders. Psychological researchers will continue to explore and look for any predisposing factors, personality issues, past traumas, social interactions, emotional problems, or family issues that contribute and could thus be intervened upon to help prevent these illnesses. And because we know that dieting and body image dissatisfaction are both big risk factors in the development of an eating disorder, we must try to do whatever we can to have an effect on a culture that continues to promote both of these. Niva Piran, from Toronto, Canada, is a prominent figure in this effort. She has shown that prevention can work. Readers should consult her work, especially her program, "Re-Inhabiting the Body From the Inside Out: Girls Transform Their School Environment," detailed in the book *From Subjects to Subjectivities: A Handbook of Interpretive and Participatory Methods* (2000): Michael Levine and Linda Smolak's recent book, *The Prevention of Eating Problems and Eating Disorders: Theory, Research, and Practice* (2005), is a monumental work and the latest and most comprehensive in the prevention area.

Various organizations, such as the National Eating Disorders Association and Anorexia Nervosa and Associated Disorders, continue to try to work on prevention efforts through sponsoring research, increasing awareness, and advocating for responsible programming and advertising. The National Eating Disorders Association sponsors a National Eating Disorders

Awareness Week, in which people from all over the country join efforts to increase awareness and work on prevention efforts as well as other goals. Readers who would like to get involved should contact this organization. Another group, Anorexia Nervosa and Associated Disorders, one of the oldest eating disorder organizations in the country, has been promoting prevention, awareness, and advocacy for a long time.

I often hear that prevention programs have been tried, but nothing definitive has been demonstrated to prevent eating disorders. However, some programs have demonstrated positive results, and these should provide the eating disorder field with the encouragement to proceed further in this area. In some cases, improvements have been shown for knowledge and attitudes, such as improvement in body image, but not behaviors. Prevention efforts targeted at people who are at high risk, for example, those exhibiting early warning signs of an eating disorder, seem to work better than universal programs, for example, a program for the entire tenth grade of a school. These targeted programs have shown some effect at changing not only attitudes but also behaviors.

In part, some of the prevention programs have not been as successful as we would like because these programs are usually targeted for very limited time periods, whereas the forces that create an eating disorder are at work on an ongoing basis. We need more programs that help girls develop increased knowledge and a better body image, like Niva Piran's program described earlier. "Full of Ourselves," a program geared to advance girl power, health, and leadership, designed by Catherine Steiner Adair and Lisa Sjostrom, is another example of an effective approach. If we continue to provide these types of programs on an ongoing basis, our prevention results are bound to improve.

In her book, *Eating Disorders* (2004), Pamela Keel reports on recommendations that were made after experts, brought together by the National Institute of Mental Health, held roundtable discussions on the prevention of eating disorders. A summary of the recommendations follows:

- We need to increase awareness that eating disorders are a public health problem and that prevention efforts are warranted.

- We need to be clear on our definitions of symptoms and outcomes to better assess progress in prevention trials.

- We need to look at basic social science research and animal research to better understand eating disorders and thus develop better prevention approaches.

- We should foster cross-discipline interactions among animal experimentalists, clinicians, and other researchers in the field.

- We need guidelines for assessing the merit of prevention trials.

- We should encourage research in biology, personality traits, family and social groups, and societal norms and values, all of which influence the development of eating disorders. Information in these areas could help us better target prevention efforts.

99. Is there anything I can do to prevent eating disorders?

The following is a brief list of what an individual can do to help prevent not only eating disorders but also harmful dieting and body image dissatisfaction that are so prevalent today.

- Do not make disparaging comments about your weight or anyone else's.
- Do not purchase magazines or watch shows that promote unhealthy dieting and/or unnatural sizes.
- Do not buy material or support shows that overly objectify females or males.
- Do what you can to help young girls learn to love and accept their bodies.
- Be an advocate for ads that show people of all ages, shapes, colors, and sizes.
- Be an activist; write letters, call people, and talk at your school or workplace.
- Confront people who discriminate and make nasty comments about other's appearance.
- Take good care of your body; this will help you be well and be a good role model.
- Focus on health, never on weight.
- Get involved in prevention efforts in organizations listed in Resources.
- Check out prevention programs on the Internet.
- Read books, such as *Big Fat Lies* (Gaesser, 1996), *Body Wars: Making Peace with Women's Bodies—An Activist's Guide* (Maine, 2000), and *"I'm, Like, So Fat!" Helping Your Teen Make Healthy Choices About Eating and Exercise in a Weight-Obsessed World* (Neumark-Steiner, 2005), that combat current myths; and give them to other people to read. These are all listed in Bibliography.
- Don't just say it and don't just believe it, but actually live your life from the position that who we are is far more important that what we look like.

PART TEN

Alternative Treatments

What are alternative therapies for the treatment of eating disorders?

- Yoga

- Acupuncture

- Homeopathy

More...

100. What are alternative therapies for the treatment of eating disorders?

A variety of alternative therapies can complement the psychological and medical treatment of eating disorders discussed in this book. Examples of some alternative therapies I have seen used with eating disorders include yoga, massage, acupuncture, meditation, homeopathy, and nutritional supplementation with vitamins, herbs, and minerals. None of these therapies are recommended as the primary or sole treatment approach, but many people have found benefit from them. What follows is a brief description of each of these modalities and their possible use with eating disorder clients.

Yoga

Not too long ago yoga was seen as a New Age trend, but now, according to a 2005 edition of *Yoga Journal*, it is big business. Approximately 17 million people in the United States go to classes and use this ancient system or set of breathing exercises and postures based on practices from ancient India. Yoga is a Hindu discipline aimed at training the consciousness for a state of perfect spiritual insight and tranquility. A system of exercises is practiced as part of this discipline to promote control of the body and mind. The postures and rituals in yoga help promote the unity of the individual with the divine. Specific postures are known to be good for certain physiological functions such as digestion, calmness, alertness, and sleep. Yoga has been studied in a variety of ways and is able to help promote a sense of calmness, well-being, and other various positive effects.

I have been incorporating yoga in my treatment programs with eating disorder clients for many years and find it useful for a variety of things, including helping clients to be in their own bodies and develop better body awareness and body acceptance. I find that this then translates to all other areas of life. A study published in *Psychology of Women Quarterly* on the Internet reported that mind-body exercise such as yoga is associated with greater body satisfaction and fewer symptoms of eating disorders than traditional exercise like jogging or using cardio machines. Furthermore, people who practiced yoga reported less self-objectification, greater satisfaction with physical appearance, and fewer disordered eating attitudes compared with non-yoga practitioners. In fact, the more yoga that was practiced in a week, the less self-objectification and greater body satisfaction there was; whereas the more hours a woman spent performing aerobic activity was linked with greater disordered eating. I believe that yoga helps people better listen to and respond to their bodies. Through yoga I have seen clients become less preoccupied with physical appearance and more interested in being aligned with their body. Both of these things help heal body image dissatisfaction and disordered eating.

Below are some quotes from my clients about their experience:

> "In yoga I found myself for the first time being really interested in how my body felt, not how it looked. It was as if I noticed it for the first time. I began to pay attention to my body in class and this helped me pay better attention to it in all areas of my life."

> "Yoga was the first time I could do exercise without trying to calculate calories burned. At first I hated it

because I thought it would not do anything, then I saw my body change. I saw that where in the beginning I could hardly touch my shins, I soon could touch my toes. I realized that with patience I developed the capability of doing the splits even though I had thought it would never be possible. Yoga taught me to be where I am with my body and myself. In fact, accepting where you are is what allows you to be happy and is even the beginning of change; I could have never ever imagined that."

"My first few attempts at yoga came when I was at a day treatment program, the Eating Disorder Center of California. In true eating disorder form, I thought to myself, 'This is not exercise. I am hardly moving. I am not really sweating. Am I even burning calories? I want to run out of this room.' By the fourth class I had a shift and a moment of awakening, ironically in Corpse Pose or Savasana. While in Savasana, tears began to fall down both sides of my face and onto the mat. Savasana is a pose of total relaxation, which can make it one of the most challenging poses. For a person with an eating dis-order, experiencing total relaxation rarely happens. I have found that either my mind was in motion or my body had to be in motion, or rest was not an option. My tears were tears of happiness. It was in this moment that I felt relaxed and connected to myself, which was something that I had not felt in a long time. No longer did I want to run out of class. No longer did I want to run away from my eating disorder and myself. Yoga allows me to experience connection on many levels. I feel connected to my breath. I feel connected to my body. I feel strength, both mental and physical. I know my body's limitations and I listen to my body. I feel at one with my breath. I am living in the moment and am fully present. I am not thinking about calories. I am not feeling fat. I am not thinking about food. I am actually living."

"Yoga, initially anyway, was very hard for me. I was a runner and was very competitive. I thought that yoga was a waste and not exercise at all. To top it off I was not very good at it, my hamstrings were tight, my back was stiff, my flexibility sucked and it was hard for me to feel like I was doing so poorly. But the teacher kept telling me that I was not doing poorly if I listened to my body, do what it needed and desired, not more. She said that if I did this, I was doing yoga correctly. I also found out that if I tried to push myself and make my body do things I would get injured, but if I persisted slowly, taking my body to its own edge, accepting just exactly where I was and not comparing myself to others, that I would improve…greatly. I began to notice subtle changes and then more drastic changes. I soon found that I could apply this principle to my eating, my weight gain, and my recovery in general and then to everywhere. I will always do yoga now. I still love to run, but yoga is a complimentary exercise and besides it is so much more than exercise for me."

Interest in yoga as a way to help heal eating disorder clients has increased over the last few years. More treatment programs around the country have incorporated yoga into their schedules. There are now a few articles written about this subject and postings on the Internet. One posted story was about a woman, Catherine Cook-Cottone, an assistant professor in the Graduate School of Education at University of Buffalo, who has developed a method of treating eating disorder individuals that incorporates yoga. She believes that yoga is useful in helping eating disorder clients find something to replace the eating disorder that does not harm them and helps them heal. Sounding very similar to my own philosophy of putting the eating disorder out of a job, Cook-Cottone says that, "As soon as you take care of and connect with your real self, that disorder will not have a job." Cook-Cottone says she already has used this approach with other eating disorder groups with "statistically significant positive results."

Massage

In the winter of 2001 I came across a study published in an eating disorder journal with the following title: "Anorexia Nervosa Symptoms Are Reduced by Massage Therapy." This caught my attention because I had been incorporating massage on a voluntary basis at my own program, Monte Nido, since 1996 and found it to be very positive.

In the study, 19 women with anorexia were given standard treatment alone or standard treatment plus massage therapy twice per week for five weeks. The massage group reported lower stress and anxiety levels and decreases in body dissatisfaction. They also had lower cortisol (stress hormone) levels after massage. Other studies have shown massage to be helpful for eating disorders as well. This warrants further study.

I have found that clients can be helped to relax with massage, and, like yoga, massage done properly can help clients begin to pay better attention to their bodies. Massage can be a way of beginning to nurture the body. Additionally, massage sometimes helps clients release information they are holding tightly in specific body parts such as their shoulders, backs, or abdomens. There are times when clients share things with the massage therapist that they have been unable to share in therapy.

Touching can be a difficult area to navigate, and massage must be voluntary. There are many considerations to make when incorporating this into the treatment process. The massage therapist must be skilled enough to handle anything that comes up during the massage.

Alternative Treatments

Several writers and health care professionals have written about touch and its healing properties. Ilana Rubenfeld has written specifically about how to combine massage and therapy in an excellent book called *The Listening Hand: How to Combine Bodywork, Intuition and Psychotherapy to Release Emotions and Heal Pain* (2007).

Acupuncture

Acupuncture is a method of treating disorders by interrupting blocked energy flows. This is accomplished by the proper insertion of needles into the skin at certain specific points, considered to be acupuncture points. Acupuncture points and the system of using needles at these points were discovered in ancient China. In terms of helping eating disorder clients, I have seen acupuncture used successfully to help with anxiety, sleep, cravings, and menstruation. I once had a client who had gained back to her goal weight, was not over-exercising, and even had brought her hormone levels back to normal but was not menstruating after eight months. I suggested she try acupuncture and within two treatments she started menstruating. Of course not everyone will have these results, but I have found that acupuncture can be a useful adjunct to other therapy. I have also seen acupuncture successfully reduce or eliminate ailments such as headaches that were interfering with the person's treatment in a number of ways.

Homeopathy

Homeopathy is a complementary treatment system in which a patient is given minute doses of substances that in larger doses would produce symptoms of the disease itself. Homeopathic treatments are supposed to trigger the body's natural healing response. Homeopathic remedies used in eating disorders might involve the use of agents to stimulate hunger or reduce binge cravings. It might also be used to treat underlying or associated issues such as insecurity, anxiety, or insomnia. However, there is no research to support the use of this form of treatment.

Meditation

Traditionally, meditation has long been thought of as a religious devotion or mental exercise to enhance concentration and contemplation to reach a heightened level of spiritual awareness. Some type of meditation has existed in all religions since ancient times. In fact, yoga stems from meditative practice. One aspect of yoga, dhyana, means "concentrated meditation." In many religions, meditation involves verbal or mental repetition of a single syllable, word, or text (sometimes referred to as a mantra). Devices such as prayer wheels or rosaries can also be useful to focus one's concentration.

Meditation is useful outside of a religious context, and in the twentieth century movements such as transcendental meditation emerged to teach meditation techniques to anyone wishing to learn. Meditation is essentially a mind-training exercise where one learns to relax the mind and concentrate on just one thing, such as the breath, or a mantra to stop the racing thoughts of the ego mind. Meditation is thought to aid mental and spiritual development but does not have to be associated with religion.

In her book, *Desperately Seeking Self* (1997), Viola Fodor has written about what she calls "quiet time." She uses this term because of the preconceived notion of meditation being connected to religion. Viola believes that quiet time helps one connect with the divine source and inner guidance, and she explains how she used it to heal her own eating disorder. The book teaches clients how to sit quietly and go inside. This can be done starting with a simple 5 minutes of silence and then gradually increasing the time up to 10 or 15 minutes. I have used this book with individual clients and in group situations. Eventually, the goal is to have clients do this on their own. Viola describes the benefits of quiet time this way:

> "Quiet time is time that we take to be with ourselves in inner silence. When we quiet our minds or suspend our logic, we allow for a quality of thinking that helps us to access our deeper being—our spirit. For centuries philosophers, spiritual teachers, and visionaries have told us solitude is the richness of self; give attention to the soul; lift the veil that separates you from your universal wisdom; and find a place of stillness so that heavenly forces can pour through you, recreate you, and use you for the betterment of humankind."

Whether I call it quiet time or meditation, I find that these techniques of going inside, quieting the mind, and becoming more consciously aware helps my eating disorder clients stop racing, compulsive, negative thoughts. It assists those with anxiety problems to have better conscious control over their body's responses to stress. There are a plethora of studies showing that meditation does in fact produce results, such as inducing calmness, lowering heart rate and blood pressure, and reducing anxiety.

Meditation along with visualization can be a powerful tool to set intentions and make positive affirmations that help create positive results. I often have clients relax and breathe deeply before we begin to discuss how they want to handle a certain situation like trying a new food. Once a person is calm, attentive, and able to focus, he or she can better produce mental images of how they would like the situation to go. The goal of meditation is not just to be able to sit still for 10, 20, or 30 minutes but to be able to bring this practice to certain moments in everyday situations. Once you learn to stop the cluttered mind and relax at home, you can bring the skills to bear while driving in traffic or hearing bad news. If you have learned just the simple skills of meditation, you can use them when you are in an argument with someone or you have a difficult stressful decision to make. All you have to do is begin to breathe deeply, focus internally on your body, and calm down. But if you have not practiced this technique, it is not possible to do it in a stressful situation. In their book, *Meditation for Ordinary People* (1999), Joe Arpaia and Rapgay Lopsang do an excellent job of making meditation easy and they explain how to begin and follow through with a meditation practice suited specifically to the novice reader.

Nutritional Supplements

Various nutrition supplements have been used with success in the treatment of eating disorders. Agents to help reduce gastric emptying or to relieve constipation are often offered. Calcium is regularly prescribed for individuals with anorexia and often bulimia to help prevent bone loss. Liquid meal replacements or supplements, such as Boost or Ensure, are used to help clients consume adequate calories. A comprehensive multivitamin is a good idea for eating disorder clients because most are not getting adequate nutrients from their diet.

Amino acids are increasingly being used for a variety of things from reducing sugar cravings to helping with attentional problems or problems with sleep. Herbs are also being used; for example, some treatment programs including Monte Nido use herbs such as valerian root as an alternative to prescription drugs to help their clients who have problems sleeping. Other agents, like St. John's wort, and phenylalanine, are being used with moderate success for depression, often suffered by those with eating disorders. Omega fatty acids are getting increased attention in treating depression and other mood-related disorders also seen with these clients. Several authors, including myself, have written about zinc deficiency being implicated in the cause or perpetuation of anorexia because this nutrient is found to be deficient in individuals with this disorder. Some studies show appetite and eating improvement with supplementation of zinc. There are far too many supplements being used to describe here, but this should give readers an idea of the ways in which supplements are used. For more information, readers can refer to *Anorexia and Bulimia: A Nutritional Approach to the Deadly Eating Disorders* (1997), which I co-wrote with Alex Schauss. Another source is the chapter, "Alternative to Treating Eating Disorders" in *The Eating Disorder Sourcebook* (2007). Both of these sources describe the use of nutritional supplements with eating disorders in greater detail.

The information described here is only a small sample of the various alternative therapies used to treat eating disorders. Alternative therapies are gaining increasing acceptance in all fields of medicine. It is important to find trained practitioners when exploring the use of alternative treatments and to coordinate these treatments with your other treatment providers and protocols.

Bibliography

Academy of Eating Disorders. *Annual Review of Eating Disorders.* Ashland, OH: Radcliffe Publishing, 2006.

American Psychiatric Association. *Diagnostic and Statistical Manual of Mental Disorders*, 4th ed., text revision. Washington, DC: Author, 2002.

Andersen, A., Cohn, L., and Holbrook, T. *Making Weight: Men's Conflicts with Food, Weight, Shape and Appearance.* Carlsbad, CA: Gürze, 2000.

Arpaia, J., and Lopsang, R. *Meditation for Ordinary People.* Somerville, MA: Wisdom Publications, 1999.

Bell, R. *Holy Anorexia.* Chicago: University of Chicago Press, 1985.

Brumberg, J. J. *Fasting Girls: The History of Anorexia Nervosa.* New York: Plume, 1989.

Bryant-Waugh, R., and Lask, B. *Eating Disorders: A Parent's Guide.* New York: Brunner-Routledge, 2004.

Carlson, R., and Shields, B. eds. *Handbook for the Soul.* New York: Little, Brown & Company, 1995, p. 85.

Costin, C. Soul lessons: finding the meaning of life. *Eating Disorders, The Journal of Treatment and Prevention* 2002;9:267–273.

Costin, C. *The Eating Disorder Sourcebook.* Los Angeles: Lowell House, 1999.

Costin, C. *Your Dieting Daughter.* New York: Brunner/Mazel, 1996.

Elisabeth L. *The Twelve Steps and Twelve Traditions of Overeaters Anonymous.* Century City, MN: Hazelden Foundation, 1993.

Fairburn, C. G. Interpersonal psychotherapy for bulimia nervosa. *The Clinical Psychologist* 1994;47:21–22.

Fairburn, C., Marcus, M. D., and Wilson, T. Cognitive-behavioral therapy for binge eating and bulimia nervosa: a comprehensive treatment manual. In: Fairburn, C., and Wilson, T., eds. *Binge Eating: Nature, Assessment, and Treatment.* New York: Guilford Press, 1993.

Fodor, V. *Desperately Seeking Self.* Carlsbad, CA: Gürze Books, 1997.

Gaesser, G. *Big Fat Lies.* New York: Ballantine Books, 1996.

Gordon, R. A. *Eating Disorders: Anatomy of a Social Epidemic.* New York: Blackwell, 2000.

Hanich, L. *Honey Does This Make My Butt Look Big?* Carlsbad, CA: Gürze Books, 1998.

Hirschmann, J., and Munter, C. *When Women Stop Hating Their Bodies.* New York: Ballentine Publishing Group, 1995.

Johnston, A. *Eating in the Light of the Moon.* Carlsbad, CA: Gürze Books, 2000.

Keel, P. K. *Eating Disorders.* Upper Saddle River, NJ: Pearson/ Prentice Hall, 2005.

Knapp, C. *Appetites.* New York: Counterpoint, 2003.

Levine, M. P., and Smolak, L. *The Prevention of Eating Problems and Eating Disorders: Theory, Research, and Practice.* Mahwah, NJ: Lawrence Erlbaum Associates, 2006.

Lock, J., and Le Grange, D. *Help Your Teen Beat an Eating Disorder.* New York: Gilford Press, 2005.

Maine, M. *Body Wars: Making Peace with Women's Bodies—An Activist's Guide.* Carlsbad, CA: Gürze Books, 2000.

Maine, M., and Kelly, J. *The Body Myth: Adult Women and the Pressure to Be Perfect.* Hoboken, NJ: John Wiley & Sons, 2005.

Moore, T. *Care of the Soul.* York: Harper Collins, 1996.

Neumark-Steiner, D. *"I'm, Like, So Fat!" Helping Your Teen Make Healthy Choices About Eating and Exercise in a Weight-Obsessed World.* New York: Guilford, 2005.

Paulson, T., and McShane, J. M. *Because I Feel Fat.* Lincoln, NE: Tony Paulson, 2004.

Piran, N. Re-inhabiting the body from the inside out: girls transform their school environment. In: Tolman, D. L., and Brydon-Miller, M., eds. *From Subjects to Subjectivities: A Handbook of Interpretive and Participatory Methods.* New York: New York University Press, 2001.

Reiff, D. W., and Reiff, K. K. *Eating Disorders: Nutrition Therapy in the Recovery Process.* New York: Aspen Publishers, 1997.

Rosen, J. *Eve's Apple.* New York: Random House, 1997.

Roth, G. *Breaking Free From Compulsive Overeating.* New York: Penguin Group, 1984.

Rubenfeld, I. *The Listening Hand: How to Combine Bodywork, Intuition and Psychotherapy to Release Emotions and Heal Pain.* Essex, England: Piatkus Books, 2001.

Schaefer, J., and Rutledge, T. *Life Without ED: How One Woman Declared Independence from Her Eating Disorder and How You Can Too.* New York: McGraw-Hill, 2004.

Schauss, A., and Costin, C. *Anorexia and Bulimia: A Nutritional Approach to the Deadly Eating Disorders.* New Caanan, CT: Keats Publishing, 1997.

Siegel, M., Brisman, J., and Weinshel, M. *Surviving an Eating Disorder.* New York: HarperCollins, 1997.

Smeltzer, D. *Andrea's Voice—One Silenced by Bulimia*. Carlsbad, CA: Gürze Books, 2006.

Thompson, R. A., and Sherman, R. T. "Good athlete" traits and characteristics of anorexia nervosa: are they similar? *Eating Disorders, The Journal of Treatment and Prevention* 1999; 7:181-190.

Tribole, E., and Resch, E. *Intuitive Eating: A Revolutionary Program That Works*, 2nd ed. New York: St. Martin's Press, 2003.

Wonderlich, S., Mitchell, J., de Zwaan, M., and Steiger, H., eds. Sociocultural issues and eating disorders. *Annual Review of Eating Disorders*. Ashland, OH: Radcliffe Publishing, 2006, p. 54.

Woodside, D. B., Shelkter-Wolfson, L. F., Brandes, J. S., and Lackstrom, J. B. *Eating Disorders and Marriage: The Couple in Focus*. Florence, KY: Routledge, 1993.

Zerbe, K. Eating disorders in middle and late life. *Primary Psychiatry* 2003;10:80–82.

Resources

Eating Disorder Organizations

Academy for Eating Disorders (AED)

60 Revere Dr., Northbrook, IL 60662
Phone: (847) 498-4274, Fax: (847) 480-9282
http://aedweb.org

Eating Disorders Coalition for Research, Policy, and Action

611 Pennsylvania Ave., Washington, DC 20003-4303
Phone/Fax: (202) 543-9570
www.eatingdisorderscoalition.org

International Association of Eating Disorder Professionals (IAEDP)

427 Whooping Loop #1819, Altamonte Springs, FL 32701
Phone: (800) 800-8126
www.liaedp.com

The Massachusetts Eating Disorders Association (MEDA)

92 Pearl St., Newton, MA 02458
Phone: (617) 558-1881
www.medainc.org

National Association of Anorexia Nervosa and Associated Disorders (ANAD)

Box 7, Highland Park, IL 60035
Phone: (847) 831-3438, Fax: (847) 433-4632
www.anad.org

National Eating Disorders Association (NEDA)

603 Stewart St., Suite 803, Seattle, WA 98101
Phone: (206) 382-3587, Treatment referral: (800) 931-2237
www.nationaleatingdisorders.org

National Eating Disorder Information Centre (NEDIC)

CW 1-211, 200 Elizabeth St., Toronto, ON M5G 2C4, Canada
Phone: (416) 340-4156 (in Toronto), Fax: (416) 340-4376
www.nedic.ca

Overeaters Anonymous (OA)

World Services Offices
P.O. Box 44020, Rio Rancho, NM 87124
Phone: (505) 891-2664
www.oa.org

Related Organizations

About-Face

P.O. Box 77665, San Francisco, CA 94107
Phone: (415) 436-0212
www.about-face.org

Body Image Coalition of Peel

C/O Peel Health, 9445 Airport Rd., 3rd Floor, West Tower
Brampton, ON L6S 4J3, Canada
www.bodyimagecoalition.org
E-mail: info@bodyimagecoalition.org

Dads and Daughters

2 West 1st St., Suite 101, Duluth, MN 55802
Phone: (888) 824-DADS (824-3237)
www.dadsanddaughters.org

Other Helpful Websites

Eating Disorder Referral and Information Center

This site not only provides updates in the field of eating disorders but also provides information and treatment resources for anyone looking to find a treatment center or private practitioner specializing in eating disorders.
www.edreferral@aol.com

www.BodyPositive.com

This is a great source of information and resources (including links to other websites) to promote a positive body image in people of all ages.

www.Mirror-mirror.org/eatdis.htm

Introductory information on eating disorders.

Carolyn Costin

The Monte Nido Residential Treatment Center, The Eating Disorder Center of California, or her new program in Eugene Oregon, Rain Rock, contact the main office at:
27162 Sea Vista Dr.
Malibu, CA 90265
Phone: 310-457-9958
www.montenido.com
E-mail: mntc@montenido.com

Glossary

Abstinence: Restraint from indulging a desire for something, for example, alcohol or food.

Apgar score: A number arrived at by scoring the heart rate, respiratory effort, muscle tone, skin color, and response to a catheter in the nostril. Each of these objective signs can receive 0, 1, or 2 points. A perfect Apgar score of 10 means an infant is in the best possible condition. An infant with an Apgar score of 0 to 3 needs immediate resuscitation.

Art therapy: A form of expressive therapy that uses art-making and creativity to increase emotional well-being. Art therapy combines traditional psychotherapeutic theories and techniques with specialized knowledge about the psychological aspects of the creative process, especially the affective properties of different art materials. As a mental health profession, art therapy is used in many different clinical settings with many different types of patients. Art therapy is present in non-clinical settings as well, such as in art studios and workshops that focus on creativity development.

According to the American Art Therapy Association, art therapy is based on the belief that the creative process involved in making art is healing and life enhancing. Through creating and talking about art with an art therapist, one can increase awareness of self; cope with symptoms, stress, and traumatic experiences; increase cognitive abilities; and enjoy the life-affirming pleasures of artistic creativity.

Attention deficit disorder: Attention deficit hyperactivity disorder (ADHD, and sometimes referred to as ADD) is thought by some but not all to be a neurological disorder, usually diagnosed in childhood, which manifests itself with symptoms such as hyperactivity, forgetfulness, poor impulse control, and distractibility. Both children and adults may present with ADHD, which is believed to affect between 3 and 5% of the population.

Biopsychosocial: The biopsychosocial model of medicine is a way of looking at the mind and body of a patient as two important systems that are interlinked. The biopsychosocial model is also a technical term for the popular concept of the mind–body connection. This is in contrast to the traditional biomedical model of medicine.

Body dysmorphic disorder: A preoccupation with an imagined physical defect in appearance or a vastly exaggerated concern about a minimal defect. The preoccupation must cause significant impairment in the individual's life. The individual thinks about his or her defect for at least an hour per day. The disorder often begins in adolescence, becomes chronic, and leads to a great deal of internal suffering.

Bradycardia: A pulse rate that is too low. Slowness of the heart rate is usually measured as fewer than 60 beats/min in an adult human.

Colectomy: Surgery during which all or part of the colon (also called the large intestine) is removed. Colectomy may be needed for treatment of different types of problems, including diverticulitis, benign polyps of the colon, and cancer of the colon.

Comorbid: Coexisting; in medicine and in psychiatry, **comorbidity** refers to (1) the presence of one or more disorders (or diseases) in addition to a primary disease or disorder and (2) the effect of such additional disorders or diseases.

Deleterious: With a harmful or damaging effect on somebody or something.

Dual-energy x-ray absorptiometry (DEXA) scan: Currently, the most widely used method to measure bone mineral density. Studies using DEXA scanning have shown that people with osteoporosis have substantially lower bone density measurements than normal age-matched people. Bone mineral density is widely accepted as a good indicator of bone strength. Thus low values can be compared against standard bone density measurements and help predict a patient's risk for fracture based on the DEXA scan measurements.

Efficacy: The ability to produce a desired amount of a desired effect. In a medical context it indicates that the therapeutic effect of a given intervention (e.g., intake of a medicine, an operation, or a public health measure) is acceptable. "Acceptable" here refers to a consensus that the therapeutic effect is at least as good as other available interventions to which it ideally is compared in a clinical trial. For example, an efficacious vaccine has the ability to prevent or cure a specific illness in an acceptable proportion of exposed individuals. In strict epidemiological language, efficacy refers to the impact of an intervention in a clinical trial, differing from effectiveness, which refers to the impact in real-world situations.

Enteral (tube feeding): Literally means using the gastrointestinal tract for the delivery of nutrients, which includes eating food, consuming oral supplements, and all types of tube feeding. The route of enteral feeding most often used is nasogastric tubes.

Iatrogenic: Used to describe a symptom or illness brought on unintentionally by something that a doctor does or says.

Labile: Emotions that shift rapidly.

Meridia: Also called Sibutramine. A stimulant medication and a controlled substance sold to people at medical risk due to obesity. Serious side effects and dependency can result from use of this medication, and it should be used under supervision of a doctor.

Mindfulness: The practice whereby a person is intentionally aware of his or her thoughts and actions in the present moment, nonjudgmentally. Largely associated with Buddhism, in which it is called *sati*, the practice of mindfulness is also advocated by such people as medical researcher and author Dr. Jon Kabat-Zinn, psychologist Nathaniel Branden, and philosopher Ayn Rand.

MiraLax: A remedy for constipation. It works by retaining water in the stool, softening it and increasing the frequency of bowel movements. It may take up to 2 to 4 days to work.

Neurotransmitters: Chemicals that are used to relay, amplify, and modulate electrical signals between a neuron and another cell.

Orthostatic hypotension: A sudden fall in blood pressure that occurs when a person assumes a standing position. It may be caused by a decreased amount of blood in the body, resulting from the excessive use of diuretics, vasodilators, or other types of drugs, dehydration, or prolonged bedrest. The disorder may be associated with Addison's disease, atherosclerosis (buildup of fatty deposits in the arteries), diabetes, and certain neurological disorders and is seen in eating disorders. Symptoms, which generally occur after sudden standing, include dizziness, lightheadedness, blurred vision, and syncope (temporary loss of consciousness).

Osteoporosis: A disease of the bones in which the bone mineral density is reduced. This makes the bones more susceptible to fracture. Osteoporosis is defined by the World Health Organization as a bone mineral density 2.5 standard deviations below peak bone mass (20-year-old person standard) as measured by DXA scan.

Outpatient therapy: Provides therapeutic intervention to individuals in need of mental health resources but who do not require hospitalization or residential care. Outpatient therapy is beneficial in providing initial assessment regarding the need for psychiatric counseling as well as offering follow-up support to individuals just graduating from more intensive forms of care. It is best suited to individuals committed to recovery because it relies on the dedication and willingness of the individual to devote to the behaviors necessary for healing and growth.

Parenteral (Intravenous Feeding): Total parenteral nutrition is the practice of feeding a person intravenously, circumventing the gut. It is normally used after surgery, when feeding by mouth or using the gut is not possible, when a person's digestive system cannot absorb nutrients due to chronic disease, or, alternatively, if a person's nutrient requirement cannot be met by enteral feeding (tube feeding) and supplementation.

Polycystic ovarian syndrome: Characterized by changes to the ovaries such that multiple follicles accumulate in the ovaries without ovulation. The ovary secretes higher levels of testosterone and estrogens. This results in irregular or no menses, excess body hair growth, occasionally baldness, and often obesity, diabetes, and hypertension.

Posttraumatic stress disorder (PTSD): A psychiatric disorder that can occur after the experience or witnessing of life-threatening events such as military combat, natural disasters, terrorist incidents, serious accidents, or violent personal assaults like rape. Most survivors of trauma return to normal given a little time. However, some people experience stress reactions that do not go away on their own or may even get worse over time. These individuals may develop PTSD. People who suffer from PTSD often relive the experience through nightmares and flashbacks, have difficulty sleeping, and feel detached or estranged, and these symptoms can be severe enough and last long enough to significantly impair the person's daily life.

PTSD is marked by clear biological changes as well as psychological symptoms. PTSD is complicated by the fact that it frequently occurs in conjunction with related disorders such as depression, substance abuse, problems of memory and cognition, and other problems of physical and mental health. The disorder is also associated with impairment of the person's ability to function in social or family life, including occupational instability, marital problems and divorces, family discord, and difficulties in parenting.

Preeclampsia: A disorder that occurs only during pregnancy and the postpartum period and affects both the mother and the unborn baby. Affecting at least 5 to 8% of all pregnancies, it is a rapidly progressive condition characterized by high blood pressure and the presence of protein in the urine. Swelling, sudden weight gain, headaches, and changes in vision are important symptoms; however, some women with rapidly advancing disease report few symptoms. Typically, preeclampsia occurs after 20 weeks of gestation (in the late second or third trimesters or middle to late pregnancy), though it can occur earlier.

Psychodrama: In psychodrama, participants explore internal conflicts through acting out their emotions and interpersonal interactions in a role play situation. The acting becomes a replacement for the typical "couch" that psychotherapists use to talk to their patients. Psychodrama attempts to create an internal restructuring of dysfunctional mindsets with other people, and it challenges the participants to discover new answers to some situations and become more spontaneous and independent. More accurately, psychodrama is defined as "a method of communication in which the communicator expresses him/her/themselves in action."

Psychodynamics: In psychology, the study of the interrelationship of various parts of the mind, personality, or psyche as they relate to mental, emotional, or motivational forces, especially at the subconscious level. Psychodynamic therapy attempts to explain or interpret behavior or mental states in terms of innate emotional forces or processes.

Psychotropic: A drug capable of affecting the mind; for example, one used to treat psychiatric disorders.

Refeeding syndrome: Occurs when previously malnourished patients are fed with high carbohydrate loads; the result is a rapid fall in phosphate, magnesium, and potassium. At risk are (1) chronic alcoholics, (2) patients with anorexia nervosa, (3) patients who have not been fed for 7 to 10 days, and (4) patients who are chronically malnourished. Refeeding can lead to serious problems and even fatal cardiac arrhythmia or seizures.

Satiety: From the Latin *satietas*, from *satis*, "enough." Refers to the psychological feeling of "fullness" or satisfaction rather than to the physical feeling of being engorged (i.e., the feeling of physical fullness after eating a very large meal).

Selective serotonin reuptake inhibitors: A group of chemically unique antidepressant drugs showing efficacy in depression, bulimia nervosa, obsessive-compulsive disorder, anorexia nervosa, panic disorder, pain associated with diabetic neuropathy, and premenstrual syndrome. There is limited controlled research on the use of selective serotonin reuptake inhibitors in children for the treatment of psychoactive disorders.

Tachycardia: A pulse rate that is too high; an excessively rapid heartbeat, typically regarded as a heart rate exceeding 100 beats/min in a resting adult.

Topamax: Also known as Topiramate, used originally for epileptic seizures but has shown some efficacy in binge eating disorder and bulimia.

Index

Index